Consumer Reports has named the cesarean section number three on its list of "12 Surgeries You May Be Better Off Without."

According to the *International Cesarean Awareness Network* (ICAN-online.org), the VBAC (Vaginal Birth After Cesarean) rate in the U.S. has plummeted 67% since 1996. According to *Newsweek*, c-sections hit an all-time high of 27.6% in 2003. According to womenshealth.org, the rate rose to 29.1% in 2004. As of this writing, the rate of cesarean births is estimated to be higher than 30%, and still rising.

The World Health Organization (WHO) states that half of the cesareans performed today are unnecessary.

The U.S. Department of Health and Human Services' *Healthy People 2010 Report* stated unnecessary c-sections take a heavy toll on pregnant women and health care resources.

Read more about these stories at the ICAN website below.

DON'T BECOME A STATISTIC!

If you feel you're being forced into a cesarean against your will, immediately contact the International Cesarean Awareness Network, Inc.:

Toll Free: (800) 686-ICAN

Website: http://www.ican-online.org

Email: info@ican-online.org

DON'T CUT ME AGAIN!

True Stories About
Vaginal Birth After Cesarean
(VBAC)

Edited by Angela Hoy

VBAC.AngelaHoy.com

DISCLAIMER

This book details the contributors' personal experiences with and opinions about Vaginal Birth After Cesarean (VBAC). The contributors, editor and publisher are not healthcare providers.

This book and its contents are the personal stories of women who have attempted a VBAC, and are provided on an "as is" basis. The contributors, editor and publisher make no representations or warranties of any kind with respect to this book or its contents. The author and publisher disclaim all such representations and warranties, including for example warranties of merchantability and healthcare for a particular purpose. In addition, the author and publisher do not represent or warrant that the information accessible via this book is accurate, complete or current.

The statements made about products and services have not been evaluated by the U.S. Food and Drug Administration, by a physician, or by any other healthcare provide. They are not intended to diagnose, treat, cure, or prevent any condition or disease. Please consult with your own physician or healthcare provider regarding the suggestions and recommendations made in this book.

Except as specifically stated in this book, neither the author or publisher, nor any authors, contributors, or other representatives will be liable for damages arising out of or in connection with the use of this book. This is a comprehensive limitation of liability that applies to all damages of any kind, including (without limitation)

Dedication

To Renata Moise, CNM, Maine Coast Women Care
http://www.mcmhospital.org/ds/services/woman-care.htm
You firm yet gentle words and touch helped me get through the worst minutes of labor, Renata. And, Mason loves your beautiful painting!

To J. Scott Flubacher, D.O.
Sadly, Dr. Flubacher passed away a few months after Mason was born. He was the only physician in our area that we could find who would accept a new VBAC-hopeful patient, 20 weeks into the pregnancy. His confidence and expertise, and his willingness to let me choose, are what made my VBAC possible. I want his family to know that he was not only a great doctor, but he was also one of the few doctors we've met who always puts his patients first. I wish there were more doctors like him!

To Andrea Mietkiewicz RN, Midwife
http://www.clearlightholisticmidwifery.com/
You gave me the courage to go for it, Andrea!

To the labor and delivery nurses and the administrators at Maine Coast Memorial Hospital
Thank you for taking care of me and Mason, and thank you for continuing your commitment to allow women to choose how they birth their babies!

And to my husband, Richard
Thank you for putting up with my moods, for constantly holding my hand, both literally and figuratively, and for bringing me any kind of food I wanted, for loving me, hugging me, and kissing me, even when I felt HUGE, and for being my rock. I love you, honey! We did it!!!

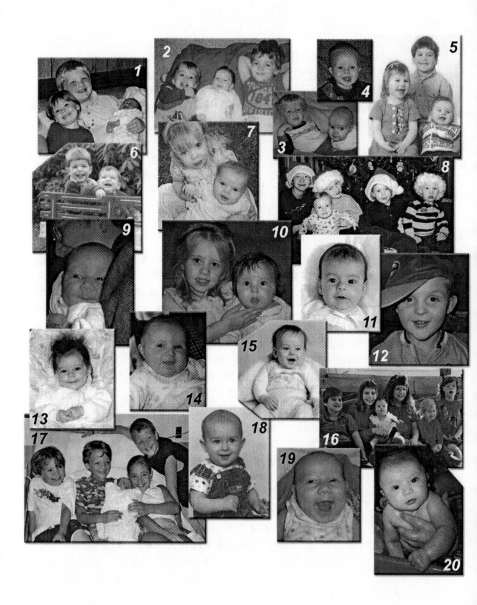

Front Cover

1. Amelia, Daniel and Abby Meritt – Chapter 18
2. Nathan, Logan and Gavin Jarmin – Chapters 21 and 25
3. J.P.'s children – Chapter 22
4. Noah Duggan – Chapter 3
5. Karen Putz's children – Chapter 13
6. Dominic and Mikolas Ruggiero – Chapter 12
7. Bridget Kathleen and Ivy Ruedell – Chapter 20
8. Brad, Ian, Chandler, Carter and Brandon Steinweg – Chapter 7
9. Sarah Kneale - Chapter 8
10. Mykaylah Anne Bean and Lydia Brooke Cooper – Chapter 19
11. Hannah Grace Duncan – Chapter 9
12. Zachary K. – Chapter 24
13. Jenna Brianne Ruggiero - Chapter 12
14. Isaac MacArthur – Chapter 5
15. Kai Duncan – Chapter 9
16. Bart, Christina, Amanda, April, Emily and Sarah Craver – Chapter 10
17. Tate, Evan, Madeleine, Lexey and Jake Atherton – Chapter 14
18. Dominic K. – Chapter 24
19. Amy Kneale – Chapter 8
20. David MacArthur – Chapter 5

Back Cover

Zach, Mason, Max, Ali and Frank Hoy – Introduction and Chapters 1 and 2

Table of Contents

Introduction
by Angela Hoy

If only...

I've said those words to myself so many times over the past four years. If only I'd stayed home when I was in labor with Max instead of going to the doctor's office so they could "check" me. If only I'd then come right home again, instead of walking next door to the hospital and getting admitted. If only I'd been more brave and not asked for an epidural. If only I'd asked questions instead of voicelessly letting medical personnel intervene in my labor, over and over again. If only I'd demanded they continue the epidural instead of giving me a narcotic. If only I could remember the next several hours of my life after the narcotic rendered me senseless. And, finally, if ONLY I'd known, when I finally begged for a c-section, how long the recovery would take, and how it would affect my next pregnancy...

But, I must start at the beginning.

I was barely 19 years old when I got pregnant with my first child. I was unmarried...but not for long! You can barely see the curve of my tummy in the wedding pictures. I went into labor at 5:00 a.m. on September 16th. My baby, Zach, was born on September 17, 1986, after 28 hours of natural, completely un-medicated labor. I was determined to be an "Amazon Woman" and I did it! Had I been better informed, I'd have been able to have him much faster and easier than I did. Instead, I starved myself for 28 hours, didn't drink any fluids (until they gave me an IV at the hospital), let them strap me down flat on my back while pushing (this actually hinders the process) and let them give me a mile-long episiotomy, no questions asked.

Zach was 9 lbs. even, alert and beautiful, and I was the happiest young woman alive.

Four years later, I was pregnant again, but this one was planned. We didn't want to find out the sex, but when they performed the first sonogram, I knew it was a girl, but didn't tell many people. She was due right after Christmas and I was scheduled to be induced on December 28th. Again, I was completely ignorant and did just what the doctor told me to do. The only instructions I refused were to meet with the anesthesiologist for a consultation because I wanted a natural birth again. But, nobody bothered to tell me how bad labor hurts when they use drugs to induce!

I woke up early on the big day, ready to go to the hospital. My husband had a hangover and didn't want to get out of bed. (Yes, we've since divorced and he gave up his parental rights in 2003.) My friend drove me, and my son, Zach (age 4), to the hospital. They strapped me to a bed, inserted the IV, and started administering the labor-inducing drug. Labor started immediately and I was in agony. This pain was many times more intense than the last time! I distinctly remember being hit by wave after wave of excruciating, unbearable pain. I screamed for help. The nurse tsk tsk'd me, telling me I'd signed a form refusing pain medication.

I couldn't take it anymore and was looking for any medical instrument that I could use to cut my wrists and end my misery. Yes, I was in so much pain, and the doctors and nurses were so indifferent to my pain that I was blindly seeking suicide to end the suffering.

I guess I screamed enough because they finally brought in the anesthesiologist and he gave me the epidural. The pain only went away on my right side. The left side still hurt horribly, but it was infinitely better than what I'd been going through. Shortly thereafter, it was time to push.

Zach pushed a stool over from the corner, put it right next to the doctor's, and intently watched his sister being born. After she came out, he said, "It's not a girl! It has boy hair!!"

Ali was born after only three hours of labor. She was 8½ lbs and posterior, meaning she came out face-up, which is a very difficult and painful way to birth a babe. The doctor didn't know she was posterior until her face emerged. She came out blue and limp. They quickly carried her to a warmer and the nurses started suctioning her and pounding on her chest and back with a funny, small, paddle-looking thing. They then whisked her away to the nursery because she was unresponsive. Our 4-year-old son, Zach, saw the whole thing and I had to pretend everything was just fine so he wouldn't be as scarred from the experience as I was.

I didn't get to hold her for two hours and I was terrified. They put her back in a warmer, and left her in my room, saying she had to lie with her head lower than her feet so the excess fluid would drain out of her lungs. So, I lay in my bed, looking longingly at my baby on the other side of the room, yet not able to hold her.

Later, an alarm went off. Her bed was getting too hot. Her temperature monitor had fallen off and Ali was being cooked in the bed. No nurses told me to keep an eye on that. I jumped out of bed and grabbed her when I realized something was wrong. She was fine and I finally got to hold her! We got to go home the next day. I had another mile-long episiotomy, which hurt like hell whenever I had to go to the bathroom (not to mention the first few times I had sex after the birth), but my recovery was quick and easy.

Thinking back, I now know that, had I let nature do its job and let Ali be born when she was ready, and not when the doctor or calendar said she was ready, these problems could have been avoided.

A few short months later, I was shocked when I discovered I was pregnant again. When Ali was only 21 months old, Frank began to make his debut.

Now, let me tell you, Frank was every woman's dream labor. I woke up in labor about 5:00 a.m. I was well rested and ready. Not only that...I was now a rebel. After Ali's birth, I was going to do things my way and nobody was going to tell me differently.

My husband (yeah, still the same guy) got up and went to work. I was left alone to labor with Zach (age 6) and Ali (21 months). My contractions were all over the place – 45 minutes apart, 5 minutes apart, 2 minutes apart, 30 minutes apart – there was no rhyme or reason to them at all, but I knew it was real labor.

Zach helped with Ali and I spent the day alternating between cleaning house and squatting in a warm bathtub. When I was in the tub, I'd turn on my Walkman® and turn the volume up really high, concentrating on the music whenever I had a contraction. When the contraction would end, I'd get up, dry off, put my nightgown back on, and do some more housework. I even stopped to wolf down two huge chilidogs for lunch. Labor starvation be damned!

Sometime in the afternoon, while squatting in the tub, I timidly checked myself and discovered I could feel the baby's head! I estimate I was dilated to 5 or 6 centimeters. That was a very empowering moment!

Around 5:00 p.m., I felt like I had to go to the bathroom (#2 as the children would say) but, when I sat down, nothing was happening. I finally called the doctor and said, "My contractions are all over the place, completely irregular, the baby is very active between contractions, and I keep feeling like I need to go to the bathroom, but nothing's happening down there..."

He firmly said, "Get to labor and delivery NOW!"

Uh, okay. My husband was home from work by then but wanted to wait to leave until he'd showered. Honestly, I was feeling so great and so energetic, and the pains were so manageable, that I said no problem. We left for the hospital at 6:00 p.m. I was just fine!

When we arrived at the hospital, I opened the car door and got out and was pretty surprised to discover I couldn't walk. It didn't hurt...it just didn't work right. My pelvis wouldn't move the way I wanted it to.

Somebody got me a wheelchair and off we went to Labor and Delivery. In the room, the nurse asked for a urine sample. I can't remember how I did it, but I managed to pee in a paper cup and put on the hospital nightie. I even managed somehow to get to the bed.

That's when I remembered how badly labor had hurt last time. I figured the pains were going to get really bad pretty soon so I said, "Drugs! Gimme drugs!"

The nurse was checking me right then and said, "Too late. You're a 9. I'll get the doctor."

What?! Nine centimeters?! Where was transition? Where was the pain? Wow!!! Now THIS was the way to give birth!!!

I looked over at our two other children, Zach and Ali, who were seated by the window. Ali was sucking a lollipop the nurse had given her. We were supposed to have another adult there to watch the children, but there was no time for anyone else to arrive. I quickly grabbed the phone and called my mother-in-law, saying, "I'm at 9. You'll never make it." She didn't believe me.

Only seconds later, the doctor was propped between my legs and I was pushing. The only real pain I felt was when Frank's head crowned. At that moment, I said, "Get it out of me!" The doctor cut me (yes, yet another huge episiotomy) and Frank slid out with ease. He never cried and was breathing just fine, and he started smiling! Yes, I have the videotape to prove it! Like Ali had been, he was 8 ½ lbs.

While they sewed me up, the nurses who'd come in to help with Zach and Ali brought them close so they could see their new little brother. I remember looking over and seeing my cup of urine, still sitting on the counter, untouched. The birth had happened that fast!

When Frank was five, my husband and I separated and then divorced. I remarried in 1999 and, a little over a year later, Richard, my new hubby, and I decided to add to our clan.

It took three months to get pregnant, which seemed odd to me. I was 35 years old at the time. Turns out I was ovulating early each month. The tryin' sure was fun, though! The pregnancy was pretty easy, but I weighed more this time around. I hit 200 lbs. for the first time in my life just before Max was born. (I've gained 65 lbs. with every pregnancy.) I also had some heartbeat irregularities that I'd had during previous pregnancies but these seemed worse this time around. Richard was a typical nervous father and waited on me hand and foot. That was nice as I'd never had a husband pamper me before!

As with Zach and Frank, I woke up around 5:00 a.m. on the morning of September 7th in labor. The children left for school and I naively assumed this time would be just like the last time, another long day of lounging in the tub and eating chilidogs. I sat on a rocking stool next to our bed and pulled out my laptop, intending to get some work done before the baby arrived. The contractions were irregular, but running around 5-12 minutes apart. At one point, I laid down on my right side on the bed and flicked on the T.V. I had two very strong contractions within 10 minutes when I did that. I told Richard, "It's time to pick up the kids from school."

He grabbed the suitcase, but I said, "No, I don't want to go to the hospital yet. I just want to pick up the kids." We left to pick up Zach (age 14), Ali (age 10) and Frank (age 8). We both got in the car and went to their three different schools. Richard ran in to get each child while I waited in the car. I had no contractions at all while we did this carpooling chore. However, I knew it was real labor and I wasn't concerned.

When we got back home, the contractions started right back up again and I knew my body was doing what it needed to do.

MISTAKE #1 – Letting the doctor's office "check" me

I called the doctor's office just to alert them that I was in labor. They said, "Why don't you come in so we can check you?"

Okay, I thought, what could be the harm? Richard, Ali and I drove to the doctor's office. They laid me flat on my back on a hard bed and hooked me up to a monitor. I had no contractions at all for 45 minutes. The nurse came in and said, "We think you have an infection. You're not in labor. We're just going to give you some antibiotics and..."

I interrupted her, "This is my fourth child and I AM in labor."

She didn't believe me.

Just then, the doctor's midwife came in and said, "Why don't we just check you..."

I was 5 cm and my waters were bulging.

Uh huh... I knew it.

MISTAKE #2 – Going to the hospital before I wanted to

They told me to go right on over to labor and delivery, which is next door to the doctor's office. I should have insisted we return home and stay there until things were further along (we live two minutes from the hospital), but I obeyed the medical personnel.

MISTAKE #3 – Getting an Epidural

We got to the hospital and my contractions started again the moment I sat down on the bed. I remembered how badly Ali's birth had gone and I asked for an epidural.

The nurse said, "But you're doing so well!"

I replied, "I want to enjoy this."

I should have listened to the nurse!!!

The boys and our neighbor, Jan, arrived soon thereafter.

Things progressed amazingly fast and I was at 10 cm before we knew it. I remember when they told me to start pushing. I remember Richard looking between my legs. And then I remember nothing happening. The baby wasn't moving down and he certainly wasn't coming out. He never crowned at all— never even came close.

MISTAKE #4 – Letting them artificially rupture my membranes

While we'll never know exactly what prevented Max from traveling down the birth canal, we do know that he was not born with a cone head, nor did he have any bruising. When they artificially ruptured my membranes, his head may have gotten wedged against my pelvis in an odd angle instead of floating into it.

Rupturing the membranes may cause the head to settle into the pelvis at an unnatural angle, preventing the baby from traveling into the birth canal.

Unfortunately, at that time, I didn't know you could refuse to have your membranes artificially ruptured. Again, I just stupidly went along with everything they told me they were doing!

MISTAKE #5 – Narcotics

The epidural quickly wore off and I was begging for relief. The contractions were strong and I was pushing with each one, but the baby wasn't moving and the pain was extremely intense and unbearable. They decided that giving me a narcotic was a good idea. I had no idea what it would do to me!

The narcotic rendered me senseless. I can remember thinking, "I can feel the pain…but I don't care." I couldn't hold my head up. It kept swaying back and forth and that scared our children. And, the drug made my face itch so bad that I clawed at it for hours. (For days afterward, my face peeled because I'd scratched it so much.)

I lost the next several hours of my life to that drug. I vaguely remember them sitting me on a birthing ball. That's about it.

Mistake #6 – Asking for a c-section instead of asking what was going on

Around 11:00 p.m., Jan, my neighbor, says I sat up in my bed, clapped my hands over my head, and said, "I want a c-section."

I don't remember that at all, but I believe her. It was at that time that the narcotic started to wear off and I came out of the fog. At no time at all did a nurse ever tell me or my husband what might be going wrong, what was preventing Max from coming out.

Our daughter, Ali (age 10), had been with me to every prenatal visit and I was very sad that she might not be able to see her brother being born. When the anesthesiologist came in, we told him our predicament and he graciously agreed to let Ali watch the c-section!

In a whirlwind, I found myself in the operating room with Ali by my head and Richard taking pictures by my belly. Ali gave me a play-by-play of the operation while she watched. She said, "Okay, they're cutting you open now. Oh, Mom! There's the baby's head!"

The doctor interrupted, "Uh, no, that's your mom's bladder..."

We all had a laugh, even me.

Then, the doctor said, "Oh my God."

I said, "What?!"

He replied, "This is the biggest baby I've ever seen!"

They pulled Max out and he was, indeed, a huge, fat baby. He weighed in at 10 lbs. 4 oz. They took him away to the nursery and I didn't get to see him for three hours. I was taken to recovery alone where a very nice nurse told me I was "all bruised down there" from so much pushing. (I looked the next day and I didn't see any bruising at all.)

My mom flew into town and, since I hate hospitals, I was able to convince them to release me after only 24 hours. I came home and began the long recovery from major abdominal surgery.

On thinking back, I think the narcotic is what did it. If I couldn't even hold my head up, how could I push a baby out? And, it was later explained to me that a baby and a mom work together during the birth. If Max was drugged, too, how could he turn this way and that in response to the pressure from my womb's contractions? He was probably just as doped up as I was.

Some may think he was just too big for my pelvis. However, he was only a bit more than a lb. heavier than my first baby, and there were no marks, swelling or bruises on his head which would indicate he was being pressed against the pelvis or stuck in the birth canal.

Now, four and a half years later, I am pregnant once again. This one was also planned and he (yes, another boy!) was conceived at Yogi Bear's Jellystone Campground in Racine, Wisconsin. While names like Yogi and Boo Boo do sound tempting, he'll be called Mason.

1. Don't Cut Me Again!
by Angela Hoy

When we went for our second prenatal visit at the Ob/Gyn's office (the same doctor as the last time), we were shocked speechless when the nurse who was looking at my chart casually said, "...and we'll schedule your c-section at 40 weeks."

WHAT?!?!

I knew I was healthy and that there was no medical reason for me to have a c-section, other than for the doctor's and hospital's convenience. Heck, I even knew about the Vaginal Birth After Cesarean (VBAC) controversy 19 years ago when I was pregnant with Zach! Haven't things changed in those 19 years? And, when I questioned her and she said the doctor would never allow a VBAC, I knew we were in for a fight...and I knew we were going to WIN. **Nobody** was going to force me to have major surgery. This was going to be **my** decision!

Richard and I returned home from the doctor's office and immediately started researching VBACs on the Internet. And, I decided to solicit help from other VBACing moms in the process. Coincidentally, as we started to research VBACs and our local hospital (which has been labeled a "VBAC Hostile Facility" by one website), our local newspaper published a letter written by the sister of a woman who'd also been denied a VBAC at our local hospital. She then birthed her baby at home.

Interestingly enough, at my next doctor's visit, the doc said I could attempt a VBAC. But, on more intense questioning, I got the impression he was just saying what I wanted to hear and had no intention of letting me go through with it. More on that later.

Below are excerpts from my blog entries that detail our investigation and our fight to avoid an unnecessary c-section, along with the days leading up to Mason's birth:

January 20th: We Had To Hire A Midwife...

Despite the fact that we have good insurance and live only two minutes from the one of the largest hospitals in Maine, Richard and I have been forced to hire a midwife[1] so we can deliver our new baby (#5!) at home. Basically, the local hospitals won't allow VBACs, even if the doctor doesn't feel it's in the patient's best interests to go through that major surgery. We feel my doctor and his nurse weren't honest with us about the situation and we had to find out information about what was really going on from other parties.

Once we learned the doctor wasn't giving us all the facts, we could no longer trust him. So, we had three choices: 1. have another cesarean because the hospital basically says they get to cut you open or you can't have your baby there; 2. hire a doctor from out of town and pray I don't have the baby on the side of the road while traveling to the out-of-town hospital; 3. hire a midwife and have the baby at home. We, of course, opted for #3. We shopped around and found a local midwife with several years of emergency room experience. She's licensed and certified, etc. and we really, really like her.

We're not getting home birth support from many of our family members. I've heard this is a common problem with other

---

[1] *We hired an independent midwife, and planned to have Mason at home, but later, after complications arose, decided to attempt the VBAC at the hospital in Ellsworth, Maine.*

parents like ourselves. Family members who don't know any better accuse you of putting yourself and your baby in danger. I suggest having some research available to show them how dangerous a hospital birth can be. There's tons of it on the Internet.

Honestly, my biggest fear is uterine rupture, but I've read that only happens in about 1 out of 580 VBACs[2]. Other than that, I think I can handle it. Lord knows, I've birthed babies without drugs before! And, if something does go awry, we're only two minutes from the hospital and, at that point, they would have to admit me and take care of us. They can't turn you away at the door if you're already in labor or if you've just given birth.

February 1st: Our Attempted VBAC Update

Last week, we went for our 20-week sonogram at the local hospital. Everything went beautifully and the baby is perfectly healthy. However while we were there, I was questioned by the woman who weighed me:

She said, "I see here you want a VBAC."

I said, "Yes."

She replied, "What did your doctor say about that?"

I immediately became suspicious and, since the doctor said we could attempt a VBAC (even though I didn't trust him when he said that), I thought he was going to get into trouble. Maybe he

---

[2] *Statistics very widely, depending on what you read, and also vary depending on the intervention used by physicians during a VBAC (inducing labor, etc.). According to our current Ob/Gyn (the one that supports VBACs), for a women who has had prior vaginal deliveries and only one c-section and who isn't given labor inducing/enhancing drugs, the chances of a uterine rupture during a VBAC are only ½%.*

was letting me attempt a VBAC and not telling the hospital because of the local controversy brewing here about VBACs? So, I replied, "His nurse told us he'd never allow a VBAC."

She replied, "But what did the *doctor* say?"

Uh oh. Now I really knew something was going on. I changed the subject. "We read that (this hospital) doesn't allow VBACs. Has that policy changed?"

She wasn't giving in. She snapped, "I don't know. What did your doctor say?"

Huh? She works in that hospital in the Maternal Fetal Medicine office and she doesn't know what their VBAC policy is? I may be blonde, but I'm not THAT blonde!

I pressed some more, "I know they used to allow VBACs here but not anymore. Do they allow VBACs now?"

She again dodged my question and only said there was a lawsuit back in 2000 or 2001 after someone died there during a VBAC. She then asked again, "What did your doctor say?"

So, I was honest. I said, "He said we could go for it."

She made a note in my file and that was the end of the conversation.

~~~~~

This morning, I once again visited my Ob/Gyn. I wanted to get his definitive word on the hospital's policy and his opinion on the matter. Before he examined me, I brought it up. We talked for about 25 or 30 minutes. Well, he talked. I listened and shook my head like a good little patient (that works the best when you're trying to get as much information as you can out of somebody).

Basically, what he said was this. The organization that governs Ob/Gyns requires hospitals that do VBACs to have an anesthesiologist and a surgeon immediately available. Does that mean in the hospital or in a building nearby? Does that mean right there on the Labor and Delivery floor? The requirement isn't clearly worded. So, while I can go there for a VBAC, if something is happening in the Emergency Room that requires the anesthesiologist, I won't be able to do a VBAC. (I was wondering…so, how would the anesthesiologist treat me anyway if he's so busy in the ER?? Hmmm….)

Likewise, if my doctor's surgery day is Monday and if I go into labor on Wednesday and attempt a VBAC, he can't drop his other appointments for the day waiting for me to deliver or need a c-section. (I was thinking…okay, so if I go into labor on any other day than Monday, a VBAC is out of the question? So…if you're so busy on that Wednesday, who's going to do that c-section?) None of that made any sense, either.

He said, "The ducks have to all line up perfectly for a VBAC to be possible."

So, I thought to myself, if all those ducks don't line up, and it looks like it's impossible that they will, he is probably going to make sure I have a c-section anyway! He'll just string me along for now, until it's too late for me to find another provider and, at the end of the pregnancy, maybe he's going to say the baby's too big or that I have some other malady that requires a c-section, just so I don't inconvenience everybody else? Is he just humoring me to get my money, hoping I won't give my money to a midwife instead? What's the point of even asking for a VBAC when it's obvious that, barring some miracle, like a parking lot delivery, I will not get a VBAC if I go to this hospital?

So, he said if the ducks don't line up, I could then refuse a c-section anyway, but then they'd have to explain the risks to me (he's already explained the risks). He also implied that you can refuse a c-section, but end up having one anyway (we heard a story that we can't confirm about a woman here who was forced to have a c-section after the doctors obtained a court order).

Basically, what he told me was that if I don't go into labor at exactly the right time, on the right day, I can't have a VBAC. It's that simple. And, the chances that all the "ducks" will line are up pretty much nil, from all the scenarios he gave me. So, in actuality, they just appear to be humoring me at this point.

He mentioned that I may have read a recent article in the newspaper (yep, sure did), and I told him I'd also read online that our hospital is a VBAC-Hostile Facility. He said, "You can't believe everything you read online."

I thought, '*You also can't believe everything your doctor tells you!!!*'

He then made a passive comment about women wanting to give birth vaginally to feel like real women. Well, I've had three vaginal births and I don't need to do that again to prove I'm a woman. However, I was still offended by his comment. I, personally, want to have a VBAC because the research I've done suggests the risks of a c-section are much greater than attempting a VBAC (something the doctor never did mention to me). And, I don't want to spend a month recovering from major surgery! At that time, I will have five children AND a business to run!

I guess he could have hidden all that information from me and just surprised me at the very end. I'll give him credit for that.

He also said if he thinks this baby is another 10-pounder, he won't let me have a VBAC. He says he would never advise any woman to have a 10-pound baby vaginally.

Hey, Doc, women successfully birth 10-pound babies the old fashioned way all the time! And, you can't use your hands on a woman's belly or even a sonogram to accurately judge a baby's size!

He actually under-calculated the weight of our last one. And, he and his nurse both told me in recent weeks that this baby was oversized (they actually told me this before the fetus was old enough to have accumulated any fat!). However, the sonogram results say he is exactly the right size for his age.

As I was leaving, they gave me two VBAC consent forms to sign. One was from the doctor's office (dated 1998, which was 8 years ago). The other was from the local hospital. Since we heard they haven't allowed VBACs since 2001, it was humorous that the date was included on that form as well. It's dated 1999. And, I wonder when the last VBAC was actually done at our local hospital...

I didn't sign the forms. I told the nurse I wanted to take them home to read. Boy, those forms sure are scary! Funny how they didn't give me the c-section forms as well. I would imagine the risks mentioned on those are much more numerous than the VBAC forms. But, nobody at the doctor's office has said anything at all about the risks of having a c-section.

I have an appointment with my family practitioner next week so he can help us find a VBAC-friendly Ob/Gyn in Ellsworth (that hospital allows VBACs) and our next appointment with the midwife is in two weeks.

Something else disturbing happened during that doctor's office visit. While I was waiting for the doctor to come in, I heard him say, very loudly down the hall, as if he was talking to someone else, "Hooters!"

I shook my head, knowing I must have misunderstood him. No way would someone who gives breast exams every day say that word in his office, and he most certainly wouldn't say it that loudly!

But, suddenly, once again, he said it, louder this time, "HOOTERS!" Then I knew I had heard him correctly. A mere second later, he opened the door and came in.

I looked up at him and said one word, "Hooters?"

He said, "Yeah, I sent some people from my office on a training trip and they had lunch at Hooters one day."

While it seems like an innocent explanation, I was, and still am, extremely and deeply offended that my doctor yelled that word twice down the hallway in his office, knowing there were women behind closed doors waiting for him to examine their breasts.

March 7th: Got the records!!!

Our primary care physician found an Ob/Gyn who allows VBACs!

After several days of wrangling, the Ob/Gyn's office finally sent my records to my primary care physician. They're forwarding them to the new Ob/Gyn this morning so we should know in the next couple of days or not if he'll take me on as a new patient.

March 8th: We have a new doc! He supports VBAC!

We received great news this morning. The Ob/Gyn in Ellsworth has reviewed my records and has agreed to take me on as patient! His name is J. Scott Flubacher, D.O.

We met with the doctor on Friday and he never once tried to talk us out of having a VBAC. He explained the risks, said, "It's obvious you've done your homework," and said my risks of uterine rupture were very low, about ½%, because of my previous vaginal deliveries and the incision (lower transverse) from my c-section. He also said they wouldn't intervene at all during the labor unless something goes wrong. That means no Pitocin and not even artificially rupturing my membranes. He said, "You're on your own."

That's exactly what we wanted to hear!

We have fired our old Ob/Gyn. I will send him the letter below only after the new baby is born. Unfortunately, if an emergency arises, I may end up at the local hospital and he may end up treating me. I wouldn't trust him to give me or my baby the best care, especially after he reads this:

March 8, 2006

Dear Dr. x,

Over the past few months, we have received contradictory statements from you and your nurse concerning attempting a VBAC at [the local hospital]. Your nurse told us late last year that you would "never allow it." On our subsequent appointment, you stated there "wouldn't be a problem." We got suspicious and started vigorously investigating VBAC's, c-sections and [the local hospital]'s VBAC history online. We learned about the lawsuit in 2000/2001 and the new VBAC practices at [the local hospital]. According to one website, [the local hospital] is a "VBAC Hostile Facility." Around this time we also read the letter to the editor in the Bangor Daily News, of which we know you are well aware.

Later, when having a sonogram at [the local hospital], the technician there questioned me about your notes stating I was attempting a VBAC. She seemed stunned that you told me I could attempt one. That, too, told me something bad was going on.

I questioned you at length the last time I saw you and you admitted that "all the ducks would have to line up" if I were to have a VBAC. You listed those "ducks" (anesthesiologist must be available and not called to the ER for something else; surgeon must be available; must be on your surgery day at the hospital, etc.). You also stated you would never allow one of your patients to birth a 10-lb. baby vaginally. Well, women give birth to 10-pound babies vaginally every single day and even sonograms can misjudge a baby's size by up to 30%. You, yourself, were off by a pound when guessing the final weight of our last baby. Basically, what you were telling me was that the chances that [the local hospital] and you would let me have my baby vaginally were nil.

A couple of weeks later, Channel 5 (whom I'm already spoken to) interviewed your partner, [Dr. S.], and his statements confirmed our suspicions. At that time, we were pretty convinced that we were embroiled in this controversy and that you were going to lead us along this path, that I'd eventually end up with a c-section anyway, and that you would have known the final outcome all along. I was even convinced that you or the hospital might even go so far as to concoct a phony reason for my need for a c-section.

You also made an offensive comment about women wanting to give birth vaginally to feel like real women. I've had three vaginal births and don't need another to feel like a woman. However, being a business owner (I'm a journalist and publisher), and having my fifth child, I'm not interested in the month-long recovery from a c-section. You also went into great detail about the dangers of VBACs but never once mentioned the dangers of c-sections.

That's also the day I heard you very loudly say the word "hooters" twice in the hallway of your office and asked you about that. You said two of your employees had been to a conference and had eaten lunch there. I was deeply offended when I heard you say that, knowing there were women waiting for breast exams behind closed doors and that we all heard you say that. I was disgusted, to say the least. I haven't been back to your office since then.

I have found a new doctor that supports VBACs and have transferred my care elsewhere.

It seems that the directors of [the local hospital] and/or your liability insurance company have been directing my care all along, not you. This is very wrong and I'm sure every one of your patients would agree with me. Unnecessary c-sections are for the convenience of the physician and hospital (and at the expense of insurance companies and their customers). While I just might end up with a c-section, it is my right to choose my own path of care, not yours, and not [the local hospital]'s. This is America, Dr. X. Nobody has the right to subject me to unnecessary surgery for their own convenience and bottom line.

I hope you will reconsider your care of future VBAC patients and try to remember that the patient comes first, not the hospital's board of directors or your insurance company.

Angela Hoy

May 4th: Only 6 1/2 weeks to go! How we're preparing.

Things are going very well. My blood sugar is under control (it's easier to manage when you're NOT eating leftover Easter candy), my weight is very stable (I expect to lose weight during the last month like I always do), I have heartburn in the middle of the night and leg cramps and I have to pee every hour on the hour, even at night. That sucks.

The baby keeps sticking his foot between my ribs in the front and my skin and it drives me nuts. My skin there either gets numb or it hurts like heck. No matter how many times I push the baby's foot down, he shoves it back up there. He thinks it's a game. Funny baby.

Max (age 4) was trying to figure out where the baby's legs were the other day (he wanted to tickle his feet), so I drew a picture of the baby on my stomach with ink, showing him head down, butt up, back to my front, etc. Max thinks it is SO cool and now wants to play with the baby on my stomach all day long each day. Today, he read the baby a book and said he would feed Mason some cookies once he's born.

After voicing my nervousness about the impending birth to my midwife, she suggested I purchase *Ina May's Guide to*

Childbirth[3]. It greatly alleviated many of my fears and really did empower me. I know I CAN do this!! I also purchased *Baby Catcher: Chronicles of a Modern Midwife*[4]. Now, THAT is a great book! I couldn't put it down!! Even if you're not pregnant, buy it.

I've since purchased two anthologies that feature natural birth stories. Most of them are hospital births, but there are a few home births mixed in.

I've decided to use the upstairs bathtub if we do the water birth and our bedroom if we don't. I labored in our bathtub when I was in labor with Frank years ago and that was, by far, the most relaxing and easy birth I've had. I can pull the shower curtain around me for privacy when people are coming in and out (it's an antique, claw-foot tub).

Everyone has been assigned their duties for the big day. Zach (age 19) will take care of Max (age 4). Max will take are of me (that's what he wants to do). Ali (age 15) will make sure everybody has what they need (food, drinks, other comfort items—she's a natural caregiver), Frank (age 13) will be the videographer, Richard will be the worry wart, and I just have to push!

Richard's pre-labor duty includes ordering and organizing all the home birth items we need (plastic sheets for the bed, etc.).

I've made a list of baby items we need. No, I haven't bought anything yet, not even one onesie. I didn't want to order things too early, but now I think it's time to start doing so. I asked for a

---

[3] *Ina May's Guide to Childbirth*
http://www.amazon.com/gp/product/0553381156/thewritemarket
[4] *Baby Catcher: Chronicles of a Modern Midwife*
http://www.amazon.com/gp/product/0743219341/thewritemarket

new cradle and a baby carrier for Mother's Day and I know Richard ordered those. We need to buy a new infant car seat, too.

My mom is still paranoid about the home birth, but at least she's stopped trying to talk me out of it. I told Richard to set up a webcam so she can stay abreast of our progress...and worry the entire time. Ha ha.

Richard's dad and step-mom are 100% supportive of our decision. Some relatives disagree with our decision while others have declined to voice their opinions, knowing we're going to do what we want to do, no matter what "society" says we should do. (And they already think we're hippies anyway because we homeschooled the children when we were RVing.)

We have 6 1/2 weeks to go. Can't be too soon for this bloated lady!!!

May 8th: Phone call reveals the truth!

As you may know from reading above, we fired our OB/Gyn after he said we could have a VBAC but then later conceded that "all the ducks had to line up" for that to happen. While he did say I could attempt a VBAC, I knew it would be impossible after he told me his conditions. We found another doctor in nearby Ellsworth who does support VBACs and we see him now (along with our midwife).

This afternoon, I was surprised to receive a phone call from the local hospital here (the one that doesn't allow VBACs—which is what caused all this trouble). The woman who called said she was calling from the anesthesia department to discuss my upcoming c-section! Can you believe that?! They knew I'd refused a c-section but they went ahead and scheduled me for one anyway!

I firmly told her that we had transferred to nearby Ellsworth because of the VBAC controversy. She asked, "So...you're not coming here at all?!"

I said, "No, we're not." And, then I hung up.

May 15th: Home Birth supplies

Last week, our midwife gave us an article titled "When Baby Arrives Before the Midwife." Wow! What an eye-opening and scary article! But, it really is something everybody has to think about.

We were able to find most of the supplies we'd need at the local department store, in the pharmacy, but other items, like cord clamps and sterile scissors, were a bit more difficult. I found a great place online to get everything else we needed (and more) at a very reasonable price.

See: http://www.birthwithlove.com

May 24th: 15 Signs I Really Am About to Deliver This Baby!

1. I haven't seen my feet...or anything below my belly button, in a long, long time.

2. After I eat a bite of pepperoni pizza, I get elephant ankles.

3. My fingernails are growing faster than my spring flowers.

4. About six inches of roots are showing in my hair (because Clairol is a no-no when pregnant).

5. My skin is blotchy and I have to pee every half hour now.

6. I am very, very moody and everyone leaves me the heck alone. If they pass by, they walk softly, fake a smile, and then walk away very quickly.

7. I am down to three pairs of "fat pants" that fit. Most of my maternity clothes, and even Richard's clothes, are too small for me now.

8. The kids no longer jump at the chance to see the baby moving in my tummy. If Mason starts moving and I call them to come and look, they sigh and say, "Ah, come on, Mom. Didn't we do this yesterday?"

9. There is a brand new cradle assembled in our bedroom...and the cat keeps crawling in there! Bad kitty!

10. There are two big boxes in our mudroom labeled "Baby Box" and "Birth Box."

11. The house is clean and, so help me, it will REMAIN clean until the baby comes and THAT IS AN ORDER!!!

12. My stomach is so big people don't even look at my face when they talk to me anymore.

13. People who ride in elevators with me have a very, VERY tense expression on their faces.

14. I took my friend to the emergency room the other day and, despite the fact that she was the one on the gurney, people kept offering to help ME.

15. And, the biggest sign that I really am about to deliver is that I asked our family physician about sterilization yesterday!

May 25th: Well, the good news is…

The good news is Mason is just fine - completely healthy in every way.

The bad news is a sonogram today showed he's in the complete breech position.

A couple of weeks ago, I wrote that his head was completely engaged and ready. However, we now know it was his butt that was completely engaged. He had me and two midwives completely fooled! No, he hasn't turned. He's been in this exact same position for weeks.

To say I'm disappointed would be an understatement. The midwife at the Ob/Gyn's office examined me today and didn't feel the head. She got quiet and I knew something was up. She sent us upstairs for a sonogram and the first thing the technician said when she put the sensor low on my belly was, "Oh, that's a butt!"

I've been patting my middle-abdomen for weeks, thinking I was patting Mason's butt. In reality, I've been patting his head. Those little fingers I felt tickling my uterus way down low were actually little toes. Those toes that have been jamming themselves between my skin and ribs are actually fingers. I feel so dumb!

Anyway, I'm going to try the exercises[5]. We'll see if they're doing anything next week when we go back in. Manually turning the baby could be dangerous and could result in a ruptured uterus thanks to my previous c-section. So, if Mason

---

[5] *You can read about breech turning exercises here: http://www.mother-care.ca/breech.htm*

doesn't turn, this will have been for naught. We'll be having a c-section.

May 31ˢᵗ: Baby Flip Flop!

We had another sonogram at our weekly check-up today. As we arrived, all the nurses asked, "Did he turn?"

"No," said I, shoulders slumped. "He's still in the exact same position."

I patted the lump just under my right rib and added, "His head is still right here. I've tried everything, from the ironing board to the elephant walk. Nothing works."

They took my blood pressure, which was a bit elevated for me (140/79). I gained 8 lbs. over the weekend in water, but lost it yesterday. That was disturbing and I'm sure glad it's gone. You should have seen my grotesquely swollen legs! They then took me to the big room to wait for Dr. F. He breezed in and said, "So, your baby is crooked, eh?"

Ha ha.

He wasted no time in gooping up my humongous belly and putting the monitor down low. He then said, "I have good news. That a head."

Sure enough, Mason's head is all the way down there, though still floating a bit (he's not engaged). The head I'd patted only moments before was his little butt.

I was absolutely shocked. I haven't felt him turn at all! I now truly have no faith whatsoever in my ability to feel where this baby is, or even how he's moving. But, thank heaven he turned!!

If I had to guess when he turned, I'd have to say it was Sunday night. I was up late in the RV on our land and trying the flashlight trick (put a flashlight down low and the baby may want to follow it). It didn't work that way. But, just for fun, I put the flashlight about mid-way up my belly, near the baby's head. He instantly got very active. I moved the light up and down, from his head to my lower belly, thinking maybe he'd follow it. I even got on my hands and knees so he'd have more room to move. He did move, a whole lot, but I never felt him turn all the way around. I thought he was just excited and bouncing. You'd think I'd notice if an 8-lb kid did a 180° turn in my belly, right? Nope. I didn't. Anyway, it was fun playing with him that way, but I didn't think it did any good. Oh, I also put some Popsicle® packages on my skin, near his head, hoping the cold would make him want to take a dive. I read online that babies usually turn by moving forward, head over heels.

I'd been experiencing severe pelvic pain when he was breech. Before I knew he was breech, I thought it was because he had a big head. The pelvic pain would come and go, so maybe he was flip-flopping over several weeks. It was gone on Monday...but I didn't think it meant anything. Also, on Monday, my hemorrhoids returned. Hmmm... And, the pinching pain between my ribs and uterus returned Monday night. So, I would guess (not that I know anything at all after all the mistaken assumptions I've made!) that, when my pelvis hurts, the baby is breech. When I have hemorrhoids and pain under my ribs, he's not breech. Hopefully, he'll keep his noggin' down and I won't have to ponder and worry about every ache and pain for the duration!

Anyway, back to the doc visit. Dr. F sat down and read the report from last week's sonogram, which was performed at the hospital. The bad news is my amniotic fluid is measuring 30 cm. That's bad. Apparently very bad. Or, it could mean nothing at all. Isn't that nice for easing my fears during these last two weeks of pregnancy?

The condition is called Polyhydramnios. Basically, I could go into labor early (I'm already 37 weeks so that's not a concern) or my water could rupture prematurely and, if that happens, there will be so much that the cord could prolapse (fall into the birth canal before the head and cut off his oxygen supply) or the placenta could separate. Oh, and I could bleed heavily after the birth because the uterus is so distended right now.

The cause could be a fetal abnormality (we've done all the blood tests and had a 12-week sonogram and a 90-minute sonogram at 20 weeks and nothing showed up at all), or I could be diabetic (my blood sugar levels were elevated a few weeks ago), or the cause may never be known. I read on one website that 65% of cases have no known cause. I'm going to keep that number in my head to keep from worrying. (Yeah, right...)

Richard and I discussed it and, because of the Mason's ability to flip (the excess fluid makes it much easier for him to turn breech again, even during labor) and because of the other risks associated with Polyhydramnios, we've decided we'll feel more comfortable laboring in the hospital instead of attempting a home birth. And, that's fine. I just don't want to have another c-section! Oh yeah, and this condition might require an emergency c-section if something bad happens very quickly.

But, the doc said today I can still VBAC.

Boy oh boy, has this boy given us some worries over the months!! Gosh, I can't wait to see what his teenage years will be like.

June 1ˢᵗ: False labor is FUN!

Yesterday morning, I was working on my laptop and crying at the same time. I thought it was because I was still so upset about another possible c-section. The more I cried while working, the more I realized it was hormones. I also had a subtle ache in my lower back but didn't give it much thought. I did have a fleeting thought that the hormones might mean Mason was getting close to launch-time.

This morning, at 2:30 a.m., I woke up with a backache. It didn't hurt much, but enough to wake me up. I then noticed a contraction starting. It was a pretty good one, much stronger than the Braxton Hicks ones and uncomfortable, but I wouldn't say it was very painful, just very uncomfortable.

It subsided and I got up to go to the bathroom. When I lay back down, I had another one. And then another, and another, and another. I was very excited, and was enjoying lying there and talking to Mason in my head, asking him, "Is this it, Baby Boy?"

Still in a state of denial, I was telling myself they were no big deal and that it wasn't labor. Then I realized I usually only have 2-4 Braxton Hicks per hour and these were coming every 5-10 minutes or so, though not very regular. I got up and went to the bathroom about a dozen more times over the next hour (the contractions were wreaking havoc on my bladder) and an hour and a half after they started, I decided I'd feel better if the suitcase was packed. So, I went downstairs and packed a suitcase with my and Mason's hospital clothes. While I was downstairs, I only had one contraction, meaning they were slowing down when I was moving around. That means FALSE LABOR. Bummer.

I was still very excited because this means the real thing is just around the corner. Could be today or it could be two weeks from now, but my body is working and practicing and Mason's arrival is imminent and no longer seems like something far, far into the future. I also had the funny thought that I'm 39 years old, this is our fifth child, and it still works!

I came back upstairs and crawled back into bed again. Richard had slept through everything, including my dozen trips to the bathroom. I'm glad because, if he thought I was in real labor, he'd have dragged me by my protruding belly button to the van and raced to the hospital.

As soon as I lay back down the contractions started a regular pattern again. I got a notebook and started writing them down. They were only two minutes apart. I wrote down the time for five of them and then stopped, knowing there was a definite pattern and also knowing it was false labor. Mason was moving around throughout the two hours, even during contractions, and I knew he was handling it all just fine. I did have a tiny bit of tenderness around the left side of my c-section scar for the last few contractions and that was a bit of a worry for me.[6] I'll have to mention that to the doc. About an hour later, I woke up, realizing I'd fallen asleep and that the contractions had stopped. That was okay, too, because I still have so much to do!

When Richard woke up this morning, I excitedly told him he'd missed all the fun. He got very excited, too. He's packing the cameras, my iPod®, etc. this morning just in case. Once we have everything ready, maybe the real thing will begin.

---

[6] *Renata later told me that having tenderness around my previous c-section scar was normal.*

June 5, 2006: Signs that labor is (or is not) coming soon

I relaxed all weekend and thought nice, positive thoughts about childbirth, and, while I think Mason turned to a backward-facing position (the RIGHT position), that's all that's happened. I've lost a few pounds (despite the fact that I absolutely HAD to have a buffalo chicken sandwich and Peanut M&Ms last night), which means he'll be here soon. But, soon could mean two weeks from now.

Here is a list of symptoms that mean he's coming soon...but none of them mean he's coming TODAY, darn-it-all:

I am having lots of contractions, strong ones, though not painful. And I'm feeling lots of pressure, meaning it feels like Mason keeps hitting me in the butt with his head, so I'm calling him my little butt-head.

My hemorrhoids have disappeared (thank you, God!) but he has not turned back to breech, so I think that's just because his head turned backwards, not sideways.

I had horrible insomnia last night. Just couldn't sleep at all. However, I did NOT feel like cleaning during that time. I had my day of nesting about three weeks ago. Other than that, I'm just sitting here feeling huge and very impatient.

I had three near-fainting episodes over the weekend, once at the store and two at our friends' house. So, I'm going to stay home for the duration. I am terrified of fainting in public. How humiliating!! And, they'd probably put me in the hospital and want to take him out immediately via c-section. No thank you! My near-fainting spells begin with my heart suddenly beating a million beats a minute (that's what it feels like anyway) and I get instantly dizzy and have to sit down. If it happens when I'm already sitting, I just concentrate on slowing my heart down and it seems to just click back to its regular beat. Weird, I know, and pretty scary.

Ali has ordered me not to have the baby this week because she has finals. If she misses a final, she has to make it up this summer. To heck with summer testing...just get this baby out of me NOW!!!

June 6, 2006: Still 1 cm and...

We had our weekly doctor appointment today. We gave the nurse/midwife at the office our birth plan for me and the post-natal plan for Mason. We're requesting minimal intervention and she didn't see any problems with our requests.

I'm still only 1 cm dilated (looooong sigh), but my fundal height is measuring 43 centimeters, which is up from 40 last week. They think my amniotic fluid level is just growing and growing (along with Mason, of course). I'm scheduled for another sonogram next Tuesday so they can measure the fluid again and also try to guess how big Mason is. However, sonograms can be off by 20%-30% so we don't have much faith in those when determining a baby's size.

They examined me and they don't think his head is too big for my pelvis. That's a relief! He is still head-down. However, they wanted to send me for another blood sugar test, a two-hour one this time, and I wasn't interested in doing that. I said, "Just tell me what you want me to stop eating and I'll do it."

We left there and got to tour the labor and delivery wing of the hospital. It is really nice. Two women were there having babies today (June 6th, 2006 - 6-6-6) and I jokingly asked the nurse if they were going to be called Lucifer and Damien. All the nurses at the desk turned to stare at me. I think Richard was the only one laughing at my joke.

Anyway, they never take your baby away from you here, even for its bath! That's exactly what we wanted!!!

I'm feeling good tonight. Richard bought me a bag of Peanut M&Ms yesterday so I guess I have to wait a couple of weeks to eat them. I made a list of no-carb foods I like (I cut back on carbs whenever I want to lose weight and there are plenty of foods I like from that regimen) and Richard (who is the best husband in the entire world!) drove to the store and bought them for me. Ali, God bless her, made me some homemade fish chowder tonight so that's what I'll be having for lunch for the next few days. I love fish chowder.

I'm working evenings now to keep caught up on my work just in case. It's actually much less stressful to work this way. I wake up in the morning with nothing to do!

June 9, 2006: Surprise Sonogram

Got a surprise phone call from the doctor's office this morning. They wanted me to come in for a sonogram at 11:00 a.m. They wanted my AFI (amniotic fluid index) tested today so they could "make a plan" if need be.

The beauty of working from home is that we can drop everything and take care of those types of things. So, we turned off our computers and hit the road. The sonogram went smoothly. Mason's head is still down. The AFI was down to 22 from 30, thank heaven!

I'm still not quite clear on what the rush was to get the reading today. Perhaps the midwife didn't talk to the doctor until today about what was going on with me this week. Perhaps they wanted to know the AFI before the full moon this weekend in case I go into labor.

25

I don't feel like labor is coming in the next day or two. Pretty quiet here in my belly. Bummer.

The children have again made specific requests about when I can NOT go into labor:

I can't go into labor TODAY because Ali has two finals and Frank has his end-of-the-year school dance tonight.

I can't go into labor TOMORROW because Zach's girlfriend is graduating from high school and we are to attend her party afterwards.

I can't go into labor on MONDAY because Ali has her last batch of finals and it's the last day of school.

So, that leaves Sunday and then Tuesday on into next week. I'd like to aim for Sunday, but I bet Mason has other plans. Richard's getting so nervous (they're doing construction on the highway from here to Ellsworth) that he wants to take the RV down to an Ellsworth campground so we'll be closer to the hospital when labor begins. That seems like a whole lotta trouble to me. I'd rather just wait and hope that labor starts in the middle of the night, when the construction isn't going on. If it is during the daytime and we get stuck in traffic, I have no qualms at all about getting out of the van, doubling over in pain, and begging the construction workers to let us pass. In fact, I think I'd enjoy that!

June 10, 2006: Labor? Nah...

With tomorrow being a full moon, and a huge low pressure system hitting us today, and all the pineapple I ate for dinner last night, I had high hopes when I had really strong and painful contractions at 2:30 this morning.

26

Unfortunately, they contractions petered out over the next hour and a half and I woke up this morning still pregnant. Darn.

June 12, 2006: 9 lbs. already? Nah...

We had another sonogram this morning and a doc appt. this afternoon. The amniotic fluid index (AFI) is still around 22, which is the same as it was last Friday and is MUCH better than the 30 it was two weeks ago.

They measured various things and estimated the baby now weighs 9 lbs. 6 oz. However, everybody knows using a sonogram to estimate a baby's size is far from an exact science. I'm hoping he weighs less than that! The bigger he is, the better my chances of a c-section.

After the sonogram, I sat up and had a HUGE contraction. It was so strong I couldn't walk. I was very embarrassed because the technician, Richard, Ali, and Max had to wait until I could walk. I felt kinda silly sitting there while everybody just waited... And, man oh man, did it HURT! It hurt so bad that I got a reminder of what labor's like and I started having second thoughts about that. But, I guess it's too late now!

That was the only contraction, though. We went to lunch and walked through a couple of stores while waiting for my weekly doctor appointment. Once there, we met with the midwife and concluded there really isn't much going on down there. I'd have to say that my body isn't currently doing anything that would indicate I'm going into labor today or tomorrow or even in the next week.

I'm dilated to "almost 2 cm." I think that means I'm still at 1 cm, but she didn't want me to feel down. She put Evening Primrose Oil on my cervix to help it ripen. I think she may have stripped my membranes, too, but was afraid to ask (sounds violent, doesn't it?). But, the baby's head is still kinda cock-eyed in there and not really settled against my cervix so he seems quite content where he is.

Anyway, maybe something will happen, maybe it won't. While we were waiting for the midwife to come in, I said to Richard, "Isn't it going to suck if we're sitting here next Tuesday and there's still no baby in our arms?"

June 14, 2006: Evening Primrose Oil

Under the advice of the midwife at my Ob/Gyn's office, I'm taking Evening Primrose Oil, which is the same thing they put on my cervix. I read online that you're supposed to take 3 to 4 - 500 mg capsules after 38 weeks gestation. Glad I read the bottle that Richard bought because these capsules are 1300 mg each! Holy cow. Shudder to think what might have happened had I not read the bottle!

Anyway, I had some minor contractions after my exam yesterday. After I took one of the capsules, I had several contractions, back to back, but nothing too strong or even unbearable, really. They just made me uncomfortable. They slowed down considerably after dinner.

I haven't wanted to go out at all in the past few weeks because I'm so big and uncomfortable (not to mention the fact that I only have one outfit left that fits, with the exception of my pajamas). For some reason, I was dying to go out to dinner last night. Richard, Ali (age 15), Max (age 4) and I all headed to Olive Garden. I was having pretty intense Braxton Hicks contractions the whole time we were there and I couldn't help but notice that Ali and Richard were just staring at me during each one, undoubtedly wondering if this was IT. I thought it was very humorous, but they did not. Seems everyone thinks I'm not going to tell them when labor begins so I won't have to spend as much time in the hospital, which I'll admit is a temptation!

Anyway, after one big one ended, Ali breathed a sigh of relief and turned her head back to her menu. I loudly grabbed the table with one hand and my belly with another and said, "Oh no! Here comes another one!"

Ali got so nervous she just about fell out of her chair. Richard knew I was kidding and we both had a good roar over the expression on Ali's face.

Later that night, I took another Evening Primrose Oil tablet at bedtime and had more strong contractions that woke me up. They stopped around 2:00 a.m. or so. I didn't have anymore this morning until I sat down to work and took another capsule. I have been having steady contractions since then. It's lunchtime now and they're pretty strong and regular, but not really painful.

Evening Primrose Oil, according to many websites, doesn't make you go into labor. It simply ripens your cervix. If these mild contractions are ripening my cervix, I'd have to say it's working.

Some websites say midwives swear by it and most doctors don't believe in it...but also tell women not to take it before 36 weeks gestation.

Now, if only the REAL THING would begin, I can get this baby out, hold him, play with him, and stop thinking about when it will BEGIN!!

Lots of people have asked me why I'm working this close to delivery. Gads, if I wasn't working, I'd be driving myself nuts wondering when the baby was coming, if he's okay, and if everything will turn out just fine in the end. Work is much better than that.

June 15, 2006: How to Gross Out the Older Kids

The only update is I lost my mucus plug last night! The good news is that means I'm dilating. The bad news is labor could still be days away...

When I told the older kids, their responses ranged from "Gross!" to "I'm outta here..."

June 17, 2006: Playing Hooky

Yes, I'M STILL PREGNANT!!!

If you detect some desperation in my typing, it's because I'm starting to get nervous. The baby is already too big and I'm terrified that, if I don't go into labor naturally by Thursday, Mason will be overdue and the doctor will recommend something drastic, like a c-section. I can't be induced with drugs because, due to my previous c-section, that would greatly increase my chances of uterine rupture. I'm not sure what choices I have other than artificial rupture of the membranes or a c-section. I guess we'll find out by Thursday if Mason hasn't arrived by then.

I had a burst of energy yesterday and suggested we all throw work to the wind, hit the road, and head for the coast (ah, being self-employed does have its perks!!). The family was thrilled with the suggestion and we all piled in the van and drove to Bar Harbor.

We ate lunch in an outdoor restaurant overlooking the ocean. Right next to our table was a railing and, on the other side, passengers were coming in from a cruise ship, and going back out to the cruise ship, via the little shuttle boat. They each had to show their passport. The cruise line was Holland America. I think most of the passengers were American but we heard lots of different languages being spoken. That was really interesting. I ate lobster (it's supposed to induce labor - it did NOT), oysters (yes, they were cooked), stone crab, clams and shrimp. I also drank a virgin blueberry daiquiri. That was delicious!

We then walked up a very big hill (it was tiring, but it also did not induce labor) and walked into lots of little shops. Max bought some chocolate rocks (they look like little pebbles) and a little train. Frank bought some gems for his collection, and Ali bought some shorts. I bought two books of memoirs about Maine long ago. Richard just enjoyed sitting on the benches outside when he wasn't following us around. Unlike the rest of us, he's not a big shopper but he loves to meander, and enjoys the outdoors.

We stopped for ice cream, ate it outside, and then went back to the van to head up Cadillac Mountain. We took one wrong turn and ended up coming back down the mountain too early, so we had to start over again. We eventually made it to the top and we sat on some granite blocks, staring in awe at the piercing blue Atlantic Ocean, dotted with islands off the coast. Frank took a little hike along the trail while Max made friends with a seagull, even telling it, "I love you!"

We then drove back down the mountain (the views on that drive are spectacular, like you've jumped into a postcard), and headed back toward Bangor.

On the way back, we smelled something funny in the van. I said, "It smells like a horse farm in here!" Richard thought it was something in the area, like all the lobster boil stands.

We kept driving and, several miles later, we smelled it again. Max was in the backseat sniffing really, REALLY long and loud. I thought he was going to hyperventilate. It was hilarious.

Richard said something didn't feel right and he pulled over. He couldn't find anything wrong so we got back on the road. Then the van started shaking a bit and Richard said it was hard to control. We pulled over immediately and Richard called AAA while I pulled out my cell phone and started trying to find a rental car. It was an annoyance but our day had been so great and carefree that nothing could put a damper on it. We kept smiling and laughing. About 30 minutes later, the tow truck and the rental car driver pulled up at the exact same moment. The rental car driver laughed when he saw we had everything in the van we needed in case I went into labor, including suitcases and even the new baby's car seat. We loaded it all into the rental car shuttle van.

We had the van towed to a dealership in Ellsworth, the same place we rented the car. They were already technically closed but they stayed open for us.

Before we knew it, we were in the rental car and on our way back to Bangor. It was about dinner time so we ate at a new restaurant in Orono. I had a big jalapeno burger, complete with salsa. That, too, did NOT induce labor.

I still have a smile on my face from all the fun we had yesterday. Clear, blue skies, a nice sea breeze, lobster and ice cream, the hustle and bustle of tourist season...what more could anybody want on a beautiful summer day in Maine?

Last night, Richard said it was good the van broke down when it did. Maybe God was looking out for us. Can you imagine if it broke down in the middle of the night on the way to the hospital instead? If that happened, Richard would truly have a heart attack and they'd have to call two ambulances instead of one.

June 19, 2006: Nice, relaxing weekend…

After our wonderful day in Bar Harbor on Friday, it was hard to get any work done on Saturday. However, I got caught up and turned off the computer for the weekend.

I took the children shopping for Father's Day gifts on Saturday afternoon. I got lots of walking in, but it didn't spur labor to begin. We went to the candy store and I got a 1 lb. box of chocolates (all my favorites). The caffeine didn't cause labor to begin, either. We bought Max a kiddie pool and I sat in the shade of one of our maple trees and watched him swim all afternoon. Richard joined me after it had cooled off a bit. We took Max inside when we noticed his lips were starting to turn blue. Even mid-June can turn chilly in Maine after the sun goes down.

On Sunday, Father's Day (Mason's due date!), we woke up to Ali cooking breakfast tacos for Richard for Father's Day breakfast. We then headed back outside because Max was having kiddie pool withdrawals. He stayed in there until early afternoon. We then had pizza for lunch and tried to get Max to take a nap with us. I'm not sure why we keep trying to do that because it never works. But, we did get some quiet time in before he was begging to go back outside to his pool.

We all went to Olive Garden for dinner, including Matt, our pseudo adopted son, and his girlfriend, Aubri. Zach's girlfriend, Sarah, came, too, so we had quite a group (nine total) at dinner and had a very festive time. We then came home, lit the tiki torches and the outdoor fireplace by the deck, and watched the sky darken over the river. It was very relaxing and the best

Father's Day ever. Woulda been even better if I'd had that baby!!

June 20, 2006: Tuesday - Lots of action, but no baby...yet

I had mild to severe cramping from early yesterday afternoon until 4:30 this morning and could even time some of the cramps. However, they eased up after 4:30 and I finally got some sleep.

I woke up this morning and am already having some mild cramping so maybe Mason has finally sent the signal to my body that he's ready. Now, if only my body would do what it's supposed to do and get down to some serious contracting instead of this whimpy cramping!

(I didn't know it at the time, but labor had begun.)

June 21 and 22, 2006: The Queen of Denial

On Wednesday morning, I woke up at 4:30 a.m. with a somewhat painful contraction. Since I'd had three weeks of off and on contractions, I didn't give it much thought. I went back to sleep.

Later that morning, my neighbor, Jan, came over. We sat in the living room and had a nice chat. During our chat, I had several contractions. They were very mild, but they sent funny shooting pains down the middle and front parts of my legs. That was odd and definitely different from the Braxton Hicks and false labor I'd experienced. She left and I went upstairs and went back to work. The pains kept coming. But, they were very manageable. They did hurt a bit, but nothing like labor pains so I assumed it was, once again, false labor. I got quite a few and even wrote them down. They were not coming in any set pattern (which is how my labor went with my last two pregnancies).

Around 4:00 p.m., I was contacted by a major news show that had emailed me and I was so excited about the potential interview that the pains stopped completely. We weren't chosen to appear on the show (they were looking for a family that RVs 12 months out the year), but I was able to give the reporter lots of information about traveling with children, homeschooling, and more.

All the while, a dormant and distant, semi-conscious part of my brain thought maybe I was in the early stages of labor. I even said to someone earlier that day that I thought Mason had sent his message to my body that he was ready, but that my body was still trying to get into gear.

After the interview, disappointed that the pains had stopped, I told Richard I wanted to go to the grocery story so I could get some walking in, thinking the contractions would start back up again. We dropped Ali off at her basketball camp game at 7:00 p.m. and went to the grocery store, which is right next to the high school where she was playing. We had Max and Frank with us. I was glad we were all in close proximity to each other. And, Zach was having dinner in Orono with his girlfriend. Orono is just a few minutes from Bangor.

As soon as we walked in, right next to the strawberries in the produce section, I had a contraction that sent those shooting pains down my legs, and I had to stop walking while it hit me. I was glad things were moving again! We spent an hour at the store and I had another contraction while we were there that also made me stop walking. But, that was only two contractions in one hour.

We left at 8:00 p.m. and parked at the gym to wait for Ali. I had two contractions while we were waiting. She came out around 8:15. We dropped Frank off at the park on the way home because he was supposed to play flashlight hide 'n seek with some friends at 8:30. We told him we'd pick him up at 9:30. I had three more contractions on the way home. They were getting a bit more painful, but were absolutely manageable and I was disappointed and kept insisting it was false labor because it didn't really hurt."

Ali and Richard kept looking at me funny and, now that I look back on the evening, they were acting very agitated. I, on the other hand, wasn't worried at all. We came home and Richard and Ali unloaded all the groceries while I took Max outside. There were too many mosquitoes so we came right back inside. Richard and Ali were making our late dinner. While still insisting I wasn't in labor, I told Ali I didn't want to eat much, just in case. I ate part of a nectarine but couldn't finish it. I later tried to eat some raspberries in cream, but couldn't finish those, either. I had started timing the contractions again when we got home and it seemed they were definitely getting closer together. But, I didn't give that much thought because, again, they just didn't hurt that much. Ali started recording them for me when she realized they were coming faster. Richard noticed, too. He'd moved his laptop down to the dining room table and was typing the preliminary "Angie's in labor" email to send to friends and family. He also got some clothes together for Max and made sure everything was in the van that we'd need.

Matt, our pseudo-adopted son, and his girlfriend, Aubri, arrived. We were all sitting in the living room watching TV. Well, I was watching TV. Everybody else was watching me. I thought that was terribly amusing at the time. At one point, I took a quick shower and didn't have a contraction the whole time. They started up again after I got out. I was still insisting, "It's false labor! It doesn't even hurt much! These are NOT real labor pains!" Nobody believed me. They just kept looking at me like I was daft.

At 9:30, Richard called Frank, who had my cell phone, and said he was coming to pick him up. Frank whined and asked for more time and Richard replied, "Mom's contractions are getting closer together. I'm coming to get you NOW." Frank didn't argue.

They got back home very quickly. It was getting late and I wanted to go to bed but everybody else wanted to go to the hospital. It was like everybody was waiting for me to figure out what they already knew - that I was in labor. I finally decided to call Labor and Delivery at the hospital. I talked to the nurse on duty, Becky, and read my contraction pattern to her (10 minutes apart, 5 minutes, 12 minutes, 7 minutes, 17 minutes, 3 minutes, 5 minutes, etc.) I told her it was my fifth child and that I honestly didn't know if I was in labor or not. I told her I was VBAC (vaginal birth after cesarean). She didn't seem at all concerned about that. I was laughing and she said that was "not a good sign." I guess most women in labor don't laugh. I was having a good time and was laughing quite a bit all evening long!

She asked if I was bleeding. No. She asked if I'd had my "bloody show." I told her I lost my mucus plug a week earlier. She said that, until the contractions come closer together and develop a pattern, I really didn't need to come in. I told her we'd time them for another hour or two and then head in if they got closer together. She said that sounded fine and that we could come in at anytime if we felt more comfortable doing that.

After I hung up, I had Richard check me to see how dilated my cervix was. I said that would be the only way we'd know if I was in real labor or not. I should definitely be dilating with all these contractions! Poor Richard couldn't tell heads from tails in there, literally (my tail, baby's head, cervix, water bag, huh?!), and couldn't tell if I was dilated or if it was my bag of waters he felt or what, so after that comedy of errors, we went back downstairs laughing.

A minute or so after I sat back down on the sofa, I had a really, REALLY big contraction that rendered me senseless. When it ended, I opened my eyes and everybody was staring at me in silence.

I stood up and said, "Okay, let's go."

Everybody jumped up and started talking at once while they headed for the door. They all seemed terribly relieved that the labor light bulb had finally clicked on in my head.

We got in the van just as Zach and his girlfriend arrived. They followed us.

I called my mom and told her we were on our way to the hospital, and said, "Everybody's *way* more nervous that I am."

She replied, "That's how it always is..."

We had a contest in the car to see how far dilated everybody thought I was. I guessed 4, Ali guessed 6, Richard guessed 7, and Frank (age 13) guessed 14.

Max has been waiting for Mason to come out for so long and he was SO excited that it was finally the day!! Then he fell asleep in his car seat. That was precious. I had the labor log in my hands and, whenever I had a contraction, I'd flip my cell phone open to see the time and would write it down. Next to the time, I'd write down how much time had elapsed between the last contraction and the current one. I'd then read it aloud for all to hear. It seems the big BANG contraction in the living room is what finally put my body on a schedule. They started coming like clock-work after that. Seven minutes apart, six minutes, five minutes, four minutes, three minutes (uh oh!)... We were almost to Ellsworth, but not quite, and the contractions were coming two to three minutes apart. I quickly went from wishing the contractions would come closer together to praying they'd slow down until we got to the hospital. They weren't unbearably painful, but they were getting noticeably stronger and more painful with each contraction. Richard, who was speeding by this time (he never speeds!), said, "Uh, at what point do I need to get nervous?"

I had just announced two minutes since the last contraction. I replied, "If they're coming one minute apart, we have a problem." Richard hit the accelerator.

We arrived at the hospital just fine, around 11:30 p.m. Ali, Max, and I walked into the emergency room and Richard and Frank went to park and get our bags. We were ushered up to Labor and Delivery (L&D) and I quickly undressed, put on a lovely hospital gown, and got hooked up to monitors. Richard, Frank, Zach, and Sarah came in very quickly. The room was pretty small... and pretty full, and I was thankful that, after all the worrying about how we'd round everybody up at the right time, everybody who was supposed to be there was there. I was surrounded by my family and I was safe. They were all VERY nervous, and I was very calm...until I realized that the contractions were really starting to hurt!

The nurse, Becky, checked me. I was dilated to three. Three centimeters!! Only three?! She called the midwife, Renata, and they determined I was not in active labor. Richard thought they might send me home. Ha ha. I told him they would never send someone in that much pain home. I knew Mason was well on his way and that he'd arrive in a few hours, hopefully by morning. (Little did we know how quickly things would go!)

The contractions came closer together and I needed my iPod to get through them. I'd crank up the volume during a contraction, concentrate on John Denver, wait for the contraction to subside, and then open my eyes to find everybody staring at me in silence. I, again, found that immensely entertaining.

Renata arrived and I was dilated to four. I wanted to sit up, but Renata said a reclining position would make it easier for Mason's head to get past my pubic bone. That sounded just fine to me! Renata was gently pushing on my stomach during contractions and that really, REALLY hurt.

At one point, I cracked a joke and Becky said to Renata, "You see? I told you she was animated." I took that to mean that my personality told them I still wasn't in active labor. I'd told Becky on the phone that I was coherent to 10 cm with my last two births. In fact, I didn't zone out during this labor until I started pushing.

A little while later, I was dilated to five. Renata had to call the surgery team in. I felt bad about them all being pulled from their beds. Renata told me she, too, had been in bed. I uttered a few apologies. She said no problem. When you're attempting a VBAC, and get to five centimeters, Maine Coast Memorial Hospital calls in the surgery team and anesthesiologist, just in case you need an emergency c-section. I admit I stopped worrying about my uterus exploding and the consequences, knowing they could cut me open within moments if need be.

They filled up the hot tub for me and I changed into my pushing outfit (a short, swimsuit cover up) and said I needed to go to the bathroom first. Everyone left the room except Ali. I walked into the bathroom and, while I was peeing, I had a really, REALLY strong contraction that took me to some other place and back. As I stood up, it hit me again and I felt the undeniable, irresistible urge to push. Oh NO!! It was too early!

I'd heard that if you push too early, your cervix would swell and, if that happened, Mason would never come out the right way.

I hugged the toilet and squatted to get through the contraction. I couldn't stop myself. I had to push!!! But, I pushed in little spurts, hoping I wasn't doing any damage, only waiting for the contraction to pass and the urge to go away. Poor Ali was outside the bathroom listening to me moan and groan, not knowing WHAT I was doing in there.

It passed and I quickly waddled into the hot tub room, knowing another one was right behind it. I told Renata what had happened in the bathroom. She said, "Well that's good!" Good? (I later asked Renata about this. She said something to the effect that laboring women who have already had a child can sometimes speed the dilation along by giving in to some of those early pushing urges. Ahhh, if only I'd known!)

Anyway, I got another contraction when I hit the water and didn't have time to ask her what she meant. The contractions were coming one on top of another then. I was conscious of what was happening but I was in SO much pain. The water helped, it truly did, but the pains kept getting worse and coming faster. What's more, the waterproof fetal monitor wasn't working right and Renata would have to push on my belly during contractions to get a reading...and I swear that made the contractions unbearable (thinking back, they were probably unbearable, no matter what).

I don't think I can describe the pain with mere words, but I'll try. I was on my back, holding onto the metal handgrips on the sides of the hot tub. Richard and Ali were in there and the others were in my assigned room. My legs and butt were pretty much floating. Renata was bending over, getting terribly wet, holding a hand-held, waterproof monitor to continuously monitor the baby. The pains would start everywhere in my belly and travel all the way down the front/middle of my legs. That was the worst part - the leg pain. My legs were shaking and I couldn't control them. Ali kept trying hold my iPod over my ears but that was difficult. I was moaning in earnest now and I was getting louder. Renata checked me. It was about 1:05 a.m. I remember there were six clocks on the wall in there and they all showed different times. I couldn't remember which one I'd looked at last so I couldn't time my contractions. I guess that was a good thing. Maybe they set the clocks like that on purpose. Anyway, I was only at 6 cm.

After that contraction, I grunted, "I might be rethinking that pain medication thing!"

I was seriously having a hard time by now and didn't know if I could go another four cm without some help. A few contractions later, the pains were absolutely unbearable and I couldn't do it anymore. I said, "I need something. Give me something!"

Renata calmly reminded me that I wanted a natural childbirth. I desperately told her that I couldn't do it anymore. I think I started crying at this point but it could have just been panicked, high-pitched grunting. I begged for help. Renata asked if I wanted Stadol. I now find it funny that I could concentrate on a conversation at this point because the pain was eating me alive, physically and mentally. But, I knew from watching *Birth Stories* and other birth shows that Stadol is a narcotic. A narcotic is what we believe played a significant role in my needing a c-section last time around. And, I remembered that the narcotic at that time did nothing for the pain. It just made me not care about the pain. And, I remembered what painkillers had done to Max. He'd been born high and didn't really wake up for two days.

I said, "No! I want the spinal thing!"

Renata said that would mean I'd have to get out of the tub. I said I didn't care. At this point, Renata said something like, "Let me just check you really quick. You might be ready to push."

She checked me (man, did that hurt!) and she said, "You're just about fully dilated. You're at 9 1/2. You can push when you feel like it."

I remember thinking 'Dang! I waited too long! If I can just ride it out to the end, hopefully it'll be over soon...'

I was relieved that I could finally push because pushing has, in my past labors, felt good and has not been painful. I got a contraction and I pushed. It hurt and it did NOT feel good. For some reason, I had my eyes open at that moment (My eyes were glued shut most of the time in the tub) and I'm glad I did. I felt a "Pop!" and my water broke like a torpedo. Boom!! It shot out of me toward the other end up the tub. You could see it under the water because it included water, membrane, and just a bit of blood. Lord have mercy, what relief!! The slight decrease in pressure was just enough to take the worst edge off the contractions. Aaahhh...

Richard ran out to get the rest of the kids and, seconds later, they were all there, surrounding me. Zach's girlfriend, Sarah, started to videotape. I haven't watched it yet, but I've been told it's quite graphic. That's good...because I didn't get to see the birth from that angle.

I pushed with the next contraction, even though I really didn't have an urge right then. Renata reached in to move a last piece of my cervix aside. That hurt, too! I was still kind of floating on my back and holding on to the tub. The pains were still shooting down my legs. I was pushing just like that. Renata suggested I put my feet in the other handles on the sides of the tub. I was pushing a few times with each contraction. In my birth plan, I specifically said I did not want anyone counting to 10 and yelling at me to push (the nurses later told me they really liked that part of my birth plan). I wanted to push according to how my body told me to push. So, I would push, inhale, push, inhale, etc., a few times during each contraction. I just did what felt right.

I was pushing while looking up toward the ceiling and Renata told me to tuck my chin down instead. I did.

It was getting more painful and Renata said, "Angela, reach down and touch your baby's head."

I had my eyes closed and, for some reason, I thought that meant the head was out. 'Hallelujah!' I thought. 'It's almost over!' I reached down and was pretty downhearted to feel about a half-dollar size circle of head and hair. Only that far?!

I pushed a couple more times and Renata told me to open my eyes and look at her. She said something like, "If we're going to do this water birth together successfully, you need to do exactly what I tell you to do."

I told her later that this was the most helpful thing she said to me throughout the entire birth. I actually, consciously thought 'Oh, thank God! She's taking over! If I just do what she says, I can get through this! My body isn't in charge anymore. She is!" Taking the responsibility of getting through the birth off of my body and putting it on someone else gave me just the kick I needed to keep going.

Renata said she was stretching my vagina and to push slowly. I consciously thought at that time that I didn't care about ripping. I just wanted this over with so the pain would stop! Pushing "slowly" be damned. I pushed with all my might!

She then said, "I think a squatting position would be best." I knew she meant was that Mason wasn't going to come out with me floating on my back that way. I immediately spun around, grabbed some handles at the end of the tub, and squatted. She was letting some water out of the tub. With each contraction, I pushed and yelled, a deep grunting yell that Renata later said was "primal." In fact, the next day, I had a sore throat. I was making a LOT of noise but I didn't care. I didn't think about other people hearing me or what other people were thinking at all. I just gave my body and my vocal cords over to nature and semi/sub-consciously rode along with the waves, not wanting to be there but knowing I had to ride the ride to get to that distant shore with my baby.

I couldn't tell by the pain or sensations, but the head was coming out. I did feel pain down there, but nothing like the labor pains. I didn't feel a "ring of fire" that other women have written about. I didn't even really know his head came out when it did. But, then Renata got stern at one point and said, "I want you to push really hard RIGHT NOW. Push as hard as you can!" I knew then that the head was out and that she was trying to get the shoulders out.

I didn't really have the urge to push at that moment but I did exactly what she said and I pushed like I've never pushed before and SHWOOOM! I felt Mason's body dart out of mine like a fish.

I don't know how but I instantly turned over and landed on my rump in a flash and grabbed him and hugged him and got my leg tangled in the umbilical cord all at the same time. I managed to untangle my leg and keep hugging him at the same time, crying and kissing my sweet baby boy. God, he was beautiful and every second of pain was worth it! I can tell you there wasn't a dry eye around the hot tub. Mason quickly started breathing on his own, making a mewling noise, but keeping his eyes closed. We rubbed him with towels and I thumped his feet under the water, but he didn't cry. He just lay there, quickly turning pink and cuddled in my arms with his eyes closed. I realized he'd slept through the entire journey!

Renata told me to put him down further in the water because he might be getting cold. I did and his cord eventually stopped pulsing and Richard cut it. (Wed specified not to cut a pulsing cord in our birth plan, too.)

Mason was born at 1:25 a.m., only 2 hours after we arrived at the hospital. Dr. Flubacher later said, "Now, that's the way to have a VBAC!"

I eventually had to hand Mason to the nurse and get out of the tub. Renata wanted me on the table ASAP for the placenta delivery, in case I was going to hemorrhage. Remember, I had a condition called polyhydramnios (too much amniotic fluid), which increased my risk. Probably 15 minutes or so after Mason arrived, the placenta came out intact. I didn't hemorrhage, or have any problems at all. I did tear but I didn't care. Renata stitched me up. Zach (age 19) came in and hugged me for several minutes. We had a good cry together. He had been very nervous when I was in so much pain and he'd been so worried about me. I assured him it was all natural and normal, and repeated over and over again, "Look, honey! I'm just fine!"

Mason was in the nursery with everybody else. They were trying to get him to cry so his lungs would really open up. He wouldn't and didn't. But, he appeared to be just fine. The nurse told me later that water birth babies are so calm when they come into the world that they often don't cry. That was nice and I was so glad we'd chosen this way to give birth to Mason.

After they stitched me up, I walked to my hospital room, where the older children were waiting for me. When I walked in the door, Frank (age 13), said, "Why are you still fat?"

When they finally brought Mason to my room after the birth, they said he was hungry. As I got ready to nurse him, Max ran over to his backpack and came back with a bag of peanut butter crackers. He started to open them. I said, "Oh, Honey, he can't eat crackers. He doesn't have any teeth yet."

Max looked very sad. He asked, "Well, can he lick 'em?"

"No, honey, he can't, not until he's older."

Max replied, "Why not? Doesn't he have a tongue?"

Not to be deterred in the least, when I pulled my nightie open to feed Mason, who was rooting around with his mouth open, quicker than a flash, Max grabbed my boob and put my nipple in Mason's mouth. The nurses roared with laughter.

I did notice later that night that Mason was breathing fast. I called the nurse in and she wasn't concerned, saying they breathe about 60 breaths per minute. Later, they discovered he was breathing 70 per minute and ordered a chest x-ray, but again, all appeared to be just fine.

He stayed in our room almost the entire time and we got to come home when Mason was about 30 hours old. He enjoyed his first car ride and he only cried when we would use a cold cloth on his butt. He was, by far, the most content baby we've ever seen. He would eat about every hour during the day (no kidding!) but I didn't mind at all. Everybody was always arguing over whose turn it was to hold him and the house was once again full of baby sounds and baby smells. We were in heaven!!

PostScript

After we brought Mason home, he continued to breathe too fast. After a few days, and a few comments from people who said it appeared he was panting at times, we started counting his breaths and were startled to learn he was breathing from 70 breaths per minute to the low 100's, depending on his activity. He was admitted to the Pediatric Intensive Care Unit (PICU). I have included this story in the following chapter. His problem was not associated with the VBAC, but it does teach a lesson about possible complications from water births.

2. A Heart Defect...or a Water Birth Complication?

by Angela Hoy

Our newborn son, Mason, was now nine days old, and had experienced rapid breathing since his birth. It was very noticeable to us and even neighbors and friends commented that he seemed to be panting at times. However, he slept well and did not seem to be uncomfortable, except when his rapid breathing interfered with his nursing, which was every time he ate.

His breathing got worse that Friday night, but we were told by the pediatrician on call that he did not need to go to the emergency room. She even had the gall to ask me, "Is this your first baby?"

We diligently monitored his breathing that entire weekend. A normal respiratory rate in newborns is 30-60 breaths per minute, but his was in the 70-80 range and occasionally in the 90's and 100's. (We were later told by our doctor that any infant who is taking more than 60 breaths per minute needs to be taken to the Emergency Room. We also later made sure the uneducated on-call doctor was contacted by our doctor about her error.)

We took Mason to our doctor's office first thing Monday morning. Max (age 4) was also with us. I was hoping they would tell me he was just fine, that we were overreacting. I felt like ice was slammed against the back of my neck when our pediatrician (NOT the one who had insulted me on the phone

49

on Friday night) gently said, "No, this is not normal. There is something wrong."

Our pediatrician told us to immediately drive Mason to a doctor in Ellsworth (who works with the pediatrician who cared for him when he was born). This particular doctor is also the doctor who reads all the EKG's in Hancock County. This pediatrician was also very concerned (you know it's bad when they usher you right into a room, ahead of everyone else in the waiting room), and sent us to the hospital next door for blood work, an EKG, and a chest x-ray. Things were moving so quickly that time was a blur. We were numb, not knowing what was happening or what was about to happen.

Mason slept through the EKG, but screamed through the x-ray and while blood was being drawn. We were back in the doctor's office in less an hour. He came into the room and quickly and bluntly told us, "This EKG is very abnormal." I felt my stomach lurch and my heart started pounding in my ears. Richard said, "Oh, God." Our world tilted at that moment and it was hard to hang on. But, we had to. We knew we had to stay focused for Mason.

The doctor explained that Mason probably had a congenital heart defect and, if it was one common defect in particular, he could "expire" at any moment. It had something to do with a valve that would instantly close and his heart would stop. Something in the blood work indicated this might be happening and the EKG further concerned him. Most babies who have this condition die by the fifth day. While Mason was 12 days old, it was not unheard of for it to happen this late.

We were now in emergency mode. Richard and I were basically in shock, veering from tears to panic and back again, and wondering what poor Mason was going to have to go through, and wondering if we were going to lose our beautiful baby boy. Oh my God, I can't even tell you what we went through in the next few hours but I'm sure some of you have probably had horrible, life-altering moments like this, too.

The doctor explained we'd have to transport him by ambulance to a bigger hospital (the one in Bangor) for an Echo Cardiogram (Echo) and, if he needed surgery, they'd have to immediately transport him to Portland (about three hours away).

He left to call the cardiologist while we sat in the room, now almost afraid to touch Mason, thinking if we startled him or if he cried, he might die. I turned to Richard and said, "If God wanted him, he would take him peacefully in his sleep. He is NOT GOING TO DIE!" I don't know where those words came from, but I somehow, deep down, knew they were true.

The doctor came back and reported that the cardiologist said it could not be one of the defects he suspected because Mason's blood oxygen levels were too high for that. So, we went from a what's-wrong-with-our-baby panic to our-baby-might-die hysteria, back to wondering what was wrong again. But, since the EKG was abnormal, the doctor was sure it was his heart.

He said, "Sometimes we get an abnormal EKG and the Echo comes back just fine."

I said a silent prayer, "Please, God, let that happen to us!"

We signed a release, waiving the ambulance transport as that would take two to three hours just to arrive in Ellsworth. The doctor said if Mason started to "expire", they would have to give him medication to make his brain think he was back in my womb. They would then use a machine to help his heart keep beating and to help him breathe. I was scared and sad, thinking Mason might have to go to sleep for awhile. Would he be thinking about us? Would he be missing us? How would he get his "num nums" (breast milk)? Would I have to wean him at only 12 days old because of this? How much pain would he have to endure? At one point would we/should we give up and say enough is enough? The thoughts and worries were coming faster than I could process them and I knew I was on the verge of hysteria. On top of that, our 4-year-old, Max, was sensing something was wrong, and was clamoring for attention.

We drove Mason back to Bangor, which is only 45 minutes away. I cried most of the way, and tried to talk to my mom on the phone. She started crying, too. She called my brother and he started a prayer chain with his church members. I can't tell you how much comfort that brought us, knowing complete strangers were praying for our baby. Mason slept and I watched his chest rise and fall, thanking God he was still with us.

We had to drive right by the house on the way to the hospital and Richard pulled up to the curb to drop Max off. Ali was waiting for him by the door. We'd called the children to tell them Mason was sick, but did not tell them how serious the situation had become, not wanting to panic them.

Richard then drove to the hospital and dropped me and Mason off to park the van. I rushed Mason upstairs. People were waiting for us in the Pediatric Intensive Care Unit (PICU). They ushered us into a room and immediately hooked Mason up to monitors, starting taking blood, ordered an IV so they could care for him if his heart instantly stopped, and brought in the Echo machine. Everything was happening so fast and I was in tears and couldn't talk. One of the residents was so very nice to me. I will never forget his calming concern and the comfort he was trying to offer. I knew this young man was going to do everything he could to help Mason get better.

Richard came upstairs at about the same time they started the Echo. It took about 90 minutes. I recognized the cardiologist as Angela C. Gilladoga, MD, FACC, the kind woman who took care of Frank during his fainting spells a few years ago. She is extremely thorough and I knew we were in good hands. I kept trying to decipher what she was saying to her technician during the test but I really didn't understand any of it. I did realize that she was teaching the technician some things during the test, and that made me feel better, knowing they were discussing the way things should look, not discussing things they were finding that looked wrong.

Mason slept through the entire test. When they were done, Dr. Gilladoga stepped in front of us and said, "There is nothing wrong with your son's heart."

I started crying again. I can't describe the feelings we had then! Such immense relief and we knew it was a miracle! God heard us!!!

They then had to look for other sources for the cause of the rapid breathing. Remember, his respiratory rate (RR) was in the 70's and 80's, and occasionally in the 90's and 100's, all weekend. They came in for a heel prick and had to get blood in a few tubes. They ended up squeezing his heel for half an hour and, let me tell you, he screamed and was purple the entire time! I kept whispering to him and trying to comfort him, but that didn't help.

Oddly enough, once that test was finished, his RR was in the 50's and 60's and, except for when he's upset, has been in the normal range every since! More on that later.

The Pediatric Critical Care physician, Dr. George B. Payne (we later found his name quite amusing), came in with the x-rays and said he thought he saw a shadow in Mason's left lung. He ordered a new x-ray for the next day. He suspected either pneumonia or a possible lung defect. We were so thrilled that his heart was okay that we were fine with a lung problem!

It was getting late and we roomed in with Mason. I was awake most of the night and I think God probably got tired of hearing me say "thank you" that night. Mason slept great. His RR was perfect and he nursed, burped and pooped often. As he nursed contentedly at my breast, I experienced waves of guilt, realizing he was eating calmly and slowly for the first time since birth, not fighting to eat and breathe at the same time. I knew instinctively after his birth that something was wrong, and I'd known every single day after his birth that something was wrong. Yet, I kept thinking it would go away, praying it was nothing but maternal paranoia. In reality, I should have never let the hospital discharge Mason after birth, when his breathing was still too fast. I should have demanded more tests because I knew, only two hours after his birth, that something was wrong.

The next morning (Tuesday, the 4th of July), Mason had another x-ray. The doctor came in later and said the shadow was still there. He was pretty sure, but not positive, it was pneumonia we were dealing with. The official diagnosis was "suspected pneumonia." I'd been praying all night, "Please, God, let it just be pneumonia!" And that appeared to be what it was!

The previous day, we'd been questioned extensively by the medical personnel about any congenital defects in the family, my pregnancy, and Mason's birth. There was some concern about my blood sugar levels because babies of diabetic moms can have heart and lung problems, and more. There were questions about my HepB status and the water birth. The pediatrician in Ellsworth told us many hospitals no longer allow water births because there have been cases of babies being infected by bacteria during the births. One baby in Maine died from bacteria during a water birth. You see, they sterilize the tubs, but the water is just plain tap water. They didn't sterilize my water. I know because I got into it immediately and it was NOT boiling!

We told Dr. Payne about this. He'd not heard of it but he researched the subject that night, and read that there have been cases of babies catching Legionnaire's Disease from hospital water systems. They collected urine from Mason to do that test, but had to send it out for the results. They went ahead and started him on antibiotics just in case. I was very happy that he listened to us and then researched what we'd discovered, just in case.

Other than his rapid breathing, Mason had not run any fever since birth, nor shown any signs of infection whatsoever. That's why nobody suspected pneumonia. Mason was moved to the regular Pediatric unit the following day and was released on the third day. We watched the Fourth of July fireworks from his hospital window.

While we may never know what happened, we do know this. Mason was born in a large tub at the hospital. It was a beautiful, gentle birth (well, except for my "primal" hollering). He was so relaxed he slept during the birth and after. He came out, did not inhale bath water, and started breathing on his own when air hit his face. He never really cried, meaning he never got that big, huge, screaming breath babies usually get after being born. His blood oxygen after birth was a bit low, around 88-90. They wanted to get it up to 94. He had a hard time getting it to that point.

About two hours later, I noticed he was breathing too fast, but the nurse wasn't concerned, saying newborns breathe about 60 breaths per minute. Later, somebody else (a different nurse) noticed it, too. They hooked him up to a monitor and he was breathing 74 breaths per minute. They ordered a chest x-ray and it was normal. They discharged him after 30 hours. We assumed all was well.

Mason continued to breathe too fast for the next 11 days. I was very concerned and worried the entire week. When Richard noticed he seemed to be panting again on Friday night, we called the pediatrician (not ours) on call that night. Monday was when all of the above took place and Monday is when they pricked his heel and he screamed for half an hour. And, as I stated above, his RR has been normal ever since that heel prick.

All of Mason's blood work eventually came back normal. We believe one of two things happened:

1. Mason had a heart defect and God gave us a miracle and fixed it.

2. Mason's lungs never fully expanded after birth, and did not expand until the half-hour screaming session he had during the heel prick.

We may never know exactly what happened. But, we do want to alert other parents to our experience in case they encounter something similar with their newborn.

Mason was released after three days in the hospital and he has been perfectly healthy ever since.

3. We Are Fully and Most Awesomely Female
by Chaleen Duggan

When I found myself pregnant at age 38, the very first thing I did was go to an OB/Gyn and request a C-section under general anesthetic. I wanted absolutely nothing to do with the birthing event. "Wake me up when it's all over!" was my war cry.

Of course, there was sound logic behind my plea. This would be my second child. The first pregnancy ended with multiple failed inductions and, after about 27 hours of labor and angst, a useless needle in my spine and finally, a general anesthetic, it was done. The best part of the entire experience was waking up when it was over. My beautiful, vibrant daughter is now six. I have always said "NEVER AGAIN". (Now I say, "Never say never.")

All in all, I can't say I was surprised to be pregnant again...it was actually planned this time. The only unbelievable part about it was that I had actually allowed myself to be talked into having a baby at age 38!! It was incredibly easy...my once declared "infertile womb" planted that seed on the first try. I refused to get too excited. I had, after all, had a miscarriage three years before and *that* was no fun at all. I figured this go around it was better to be low-key. With my health issues, it seemed the prudent thing to do. How wonderful it would be if all pregnancies were approached with a positive attitude and encouragement!

Being an old girl, pushing 38, and having lung disease to boot, along with a host of other autoimmune issues, I was not exactly what you would call prime breeding stock. Sure, I might be witty, intelligent and attractive, but those traits are irrelevant when one is reviewing the merits of a womb.

My health was the main issue of my pregnancy from the beginning. I had lost a baby at 3½ months a couple years before. That paired up with the pregnancy and/or delivery of my beautiful daughter left me having serious doubts about my ability to be able to "grow a baby"... and I had a complete lack of confidence in myself in this regard.

So, I did nothing. I knew I was pregnant, but I fully expected this little one would not make it, so I did not tell anyone. I did not get excited. I did not make grand plans. I knew, in my heart, it was a boy, but I did not listen for him. With my daughter, I knew her from the first week, growing safe in my belly. I spoke to her. She let me know her name. It was all so mystical and perfect (aside from the harsh reality of perpetual nausea). I knew with the first one I was going to have a baby. And I did.

During the first pregnancy, I was always looking at babies' heads, thinking to myself "man that has got to hurt!" I would visibly shudder every time I saw a big old melon on a wee baby. When it came down to the big push... I held back. I was a complete mess after multiple attempts at induction and having had my water broken the morning before, and then there was the 27 hours of labor. I was exhausted and nobody would feed me, which did not help my disposition at all. I had read that sometimes when you push you poop, and I was mortified to poop in plain view of people, or worse yet on my baby, so I held back.

There was this one nurse who had a wonky eye. She seemed to take a real interest in me. Any excuse she happened upon, she would state she had to examine me. Those people examined me repeatedly over the course of 27 hours. It hurt. It felt like rape. I wasn't sure what the point of all the poking and prodding was, but it didn't help my attitude OR the labor at all. These were the memories I had of my first labor and I vowed then and there the second time around would be different!

I finally went in to see an OB/Gyn close to my fourth month. By that time, I still was not gaining any weight and I figured it was time to find out if there was going to be a baby at all. Nature has a way of figuring all this stuff out if we just allow it to happen. Well, it turned out I was indeed pregnant, and even though I had lost weight and the educated folk were gravely concerned and even questioning the wisdom of following through with this "high-risk" pregnancy (a subtle way of suggesting termination), the ultrasound showed a very healthy, perfectly formed, nice-sized boy. I ignored their hints and looks of doom and continued to be pregnant, trying to relax and be happy and look forward to this little person who was growing inside me and ruining my taste for meat and ginger ale

I couldn't get off the couch if my life depended on it most days. My right side was excruciating. I think they call that sciatica but I was afraid to say anything. They might have tried to convince me in a moment of weakness to have a c-section or something.

I realized that because of my age and health, I was being treated like a sickly patient (and a lousy one at that, because I had DARED to get pregnant in my condition). At age 38 and disabled with a lung condition, I was "geriatric" and "high-risk." The knowledgeable professionals stated on more than one occasion that I was not gaining and the baby might have to be taken early for his own benefit. (The resulting ultrasound showed the baby to be a week ahead for size, which served to put an end to THAT particular fear-instilling nonsense.) I was booked for consult after consult, and because of my rural location I had to drive two hours round trip to each appointment. I made every effort to be a compliant patient. One week, towards our due date, I had to drive that two-hour trip four times in blistering heat with no air conditioning. Every doctor said the same thing, "Bed Rest, Bed Rest, Bed Rest."

And, I would reply, "That is exactly where I would be if I was not spending my day in your office!"

Not that I minded the office waits. I have spent plenty of time in waiting rooms for tests or consults for my lungs. In fact, I was the first one to defend the obstetrician when he had to leave in the middle of the day to go to the hospital. The complaints had to be addressed, and I remember not so long ago it was *me* he had come to assist, thereby leaving a room full of pregnant ladies twitching and groaning. I would always point out that we were safe in the waiting room, and wouldn't we rather be here waiting than over there, at the hospital, in the middle of a miscarriage or some other crisis? I know this because three years before it had been me. No, it wasn't the waiting…it was the sign, "NO FOOD OR DRINKS." That is what I really hated. I can sit anywhere for five hours but, for God's sake, don't starve me!

So I waltzed into his office one day about a week before the c-section was booked and made my announcement. Can you imagine their outrage, after the many efforts they made to "manage" me, when out of the blue I announced I was no longer a patient but pregnant woman, and I had changed my mind. I was going to have this baby the old-fashioned way. No c-section, no drugs. In fact, I didn't even want anyone in the room! This experience was between me and the baby and "the Big Guy" up above.

The doctor gave me a look as if to say "Yeah, right. I've heard this before." And, then he suggested we keep the day booked anyway just in case I changed my mind again. He reminded me that childbirth hurts. Well, yeah, when you examine the physics of it, I GUESS SO! I told him I live in a world of pain, what were a few extra hours? MY MY MY, we are so cocky when we think we have the tiger by the tail.

> *I realized all at once that I had allowed the medical community to micro-manage me.*

By the last eight weeks, I was gaining two pounds a week. I made the mistake of picking up a watermelon at the grocers and I awoke later that night. WOW! My leg felt like it was tied in a pretzel....sciatica!

I was busy trying to figure out how all this running around to different doctors was helping with the prescribed bed-rest...when one morning between the tea and toothpaste, I had an epiphany. I realized all at once that I had allowed the medical community to micro-manage me. I was being treated like a sick patient, not a pregnant lady. The result being that I had completely lost faith in my body's ability to perform the task nature had designed it for. My previous experience had assisted in this outcome.

I had to take the time, sit down, and give this whole thing the consideration it deserved. I had to ask the questions: "Why was I so agreeable to a c-section in the first place...had in fact waltzed in and demanded one? Why was I so fearful of labor? What needed to happen for me to be able to reconsider this thing? What were my incentives to do this thing the way God intended?

I had to remove the authority from the external sources and give it back to my "self", for my lack of faith in my body must surely be received on some internal level as an insult!

Medical technology is an awesome compliment to Mother Nature...but if we don't take responsibility for our own self, it threatens to replace nature. The line can be hard to find (until we trip over it), unless we are looking for it.

I guess I just woke up one day and decided this was MY experience and I was gong to do it MY WAY. When I told the doctors my decision, they didn't seem to put much stock in it. "Well, let's keep the c-section booked in case you change your mind", and of course I agreed just to keep them happy...and quiet.

I had decided immediately I did not want a group of people there. I did not need a cheering committee, nor did I need a bunch of people looking at my privates, or pretending they could see a head when there was nothing...I had been through all this before and it wasn't going to be my story again.

Towards the end of my term, actually what turned out to be two days before my labor began, I made it up to the appointment for my blood work and pre-admission clinic for the c-section. I listened with half an ear, trying to look interested when finally the +118 degree F humidity got to me, and I told the nurse, "There is something you should know. All this is very interesting, and I have every intention of being a compliant patient...but um, I have changed my mind on the whole c-section thing."

"What are you saying?"

"Well. I have decided I am going to have this baby the way God intended. I don't want to waste any more of your valuable time. I just thought you should know."

She looked at me with raw disbelief. I could almost SEE what she was thinking. She put on her poker face and wrote something in my chart and said, "You're sure, right? You do have a space booked in the Operating Room for a c-section and a tubal ligation..."

I stopped her right there. "NOPE. I am done with being treated like a sick patient. I am a pregnant woman and that is how I wish to be treated. This is not a disease I have, but a gift I carry. Women have been having babies the 'hard way' ever since the beginning of time. That is how we were designed. I am prepared to try. If there are problems, then it is good to know there is an option."

"Okay, well.... I took the liberty of booking you in for an anesthetic consult. When you leave here, go over to the other site and...blah blah blah..."

I was sure she had heard nothing and had just shrugged off my decision as pre-push jitters?

GOSH it was hot.

I made my way over to the other site, paid another $3.00 for parking, thinking this was some gig where the nurses get a cut of the parking fees, and went up to see the doctor who was going to put me to sleep for the c-section...or who THOUGHT he was going to.

Of all the docs, he was the only one who suggested that, due to my health, I would be better off going natural. His reason was similar; he did not want to be sued. He did not want anything to do with a patient with pulmonary issues in his operating theatre. He was honest about that. He assured me that it would not take two hours to get a team to the Operating Room. It would take about 20 minutes. He looked relieved and wished me the best of luck.

It was like permission.

The next day, I was back in the city, another hour drive. It was incredibly hot and humid but I couldn't let my people down. I

63

was the president of our town's Horticultural Society and I had to pick up the annual plantings for the town gardens. We had scheduled a huge "planting marathon" for the next morning. All the town gardens were to be planted. By then, I was 39 weeks pregnant and feeling every week of it in the form of a 3-inch nail in my back. I loaded up the car with trays and trays of pretty flowers and drove the hour back home.

The next morning, we all gathered early, before it became too insanely hot, and started planting. It went smoothly. We drove to each park and loaded up the planters. It was a relaxing, fun day, yet there was the feeling of hurry. The rush was to finish before it became too hot. By 10 a.m., it was above 90 and the humidity was making it hard to breath. My companions kept nagging me to sit and not carry anything and rest and...ack!

I kept telling them, "Well I am having my baby this weekend. I have it all planned. I need to exert myself in order to encourage him!"

We managed to finish the last planter around 2:30 p.m. It was starting to cloud over and there was thunder in the distance - very ominous. Living in this region, on the banks of a river that has a mountain on one side, we get every weather system around. Nothing passes unnoticed.

I dragged my weary bump home with my five-year-old and we crawled into a warm tub. By 3 p.m., we were both in bed, asleep. Around 6 p.m., I woke up. There was no electricity. It was eerie. It was so quiet out there...and dark. The storm had passed but it was still so dark! The first thing I noticed was the sheets seemed damp. I had apparently peed the bed. "Oh, great! Not only am I clumsy and limping from sciatica, now I am also incontinent!" A trip to the can reassured me that I was perfectly able to hold my bladder. It was then that I concluded I might be starting labor.

Funny thing, labor... You just never know how it's all gonna go down.

I had no pain, no twinge, no wracking, bone-scraping sensations....just a periodic trickle.

Well it took about 45 minutes to find a phone that would work without power and the first person I called was my cousin in the city.

"Oh, hi. How are you? Did you get that storm? I think I am in labor, so how about those Blue Jays, eh?" or something like that. Ha ha. She hung up on me when I got to the ballgame part, right after suggesting I get my bony hide into the hospital.

The next call was to my sitter (my five-year-old was still blissfully ignorant and sleeping - she worked hard in those gardens). "I think it is time." Then I went and packed some clothes for my daughter.

Finally, it was time to call for my ride. I was hungry but nothing was open. I guess the power had been out for hours, so I did not want to open the fridge to snack for fear of spoiling any food.

It was no great concern because I figured we could eat in North Bay. I knew one thing for sure and that was, this time I was planning ahead. I knew exactly what I was going to sneak into labor and delivery because GOD KNOWS they starve you once you get in there.

So my driver picked us up and we dropped off the weary child, and headed for the city. The first stop was for FOOD. I had taken care of the trickling issue with a monster pad and I was prepared to risk a flood or whatever it took, but I was NOT going to that hospital on an empty stomach. So we drove around looking for a place to eat. As luck would have it, every place we went past was closed. Obviously, they had the same storm because there was no power in the city, either, just small patches of lights here and there. The fast food place (Wendy's®) was an oasis. I waddled in and wasted no time deciding that I had to have a Biggie this and a Biggie that and then I went to sit down. I was feeling a little funny every once in a while. It was hormones or an odd twinge, but most of all I was hungry.

So my driver was standing there ordering my lumberjack meal while I sat waiting in a booth in that incredible heat. I am not sure if I looked odd but I must have because a man approached me and asked if I was okay.

"Yes, I am fine, thank you."

"Oh, well, you don't look so good"

"Oh that. I am in labor. My water broke and I feel a little strange, but I'm really just fine! No worries"

He steps back, incredulous.

"Labor?!? Shouldn't you be on your way to the hospital?!"

"Oh yes, we are heading there next. The thing is, see, I am not going in there on an empty stomach. THEY STARVE YOU IN THAT PLACE!"

"Really?!?! You're serious?"

I nodded emphatically, "Oh yes, I have to go through a marathon tonight and I need my Wheaties®. Try to explain THAT to a bossy nurse!"

He stood there for a moment, then nodded and said, "Well the best of luck to you!" and went on to order his Spicy Chicken Combo®. I caught him glancing at me a couple times. He seemed nervous. He did not stay to eat.

~~~

The first thing they asked me at the hospital was when my water broke. They have this idea that if you don't get that baby pushed out within 24 hours of the water breaking you HAVE to have a c-section. It has to do with an increased risk of infection or something. Not sure who came up with the magic number - "24" - but I DO know that in Canada, OB/Gyn guys are paid by the delivery, not the hour, and I strongly suspected this had something to do with it, too.

Therefore, I told them what I believed to be the truth.

You see, it was now 11 p.m., and they were questioning my sanity, I suppose, showing up hours after I had called the labor unit with two bags of fast food and a huge cup of iced tea.

"Well, I woke up to a trickle at 6 p.m."

"So...it broke BEFORE that..."

"NO. I WOKE UP to the trickle."

"Well, then, how do you know when it broke?! You were asleep."

Me, thinking quickly now, having a flashback to my troubled youth and the nuns...my greatest fear, getting caught in a lie... "No I did not pass a note in science class, sister." "Because the sheets were dry." The nurse nodded. (Phew! No detention!)

I knew that if I went in there with the attitude that my body could do this, if I refused to listen to the dubious negativity and the offers of an easy-out, that my body could do this. I was not giving my "self" the chance! My decision had initially been based on fear…and I realized it didn't have to be that way.

"Oh, so you are booked for a c-section. We'll call the OB."

"Um…no. I want the trial of labor."

"Have you discussed this with your doctor?"

"I mentioned it to him. I discussed it with my baby, though, and he seems to be all for it."

Boy, they just loved me.

At that point, I noticed my bedside table with all the food on it had been moved over a foot or so…AWAY from me.

"So, how do you KNOW your water broke? Maybe it was something else."

"Um…I know it broke because I am leaking."

"Well we have no idea if it is amniotic fluid. We'll have to do a swab."

"Listen. NOBODY is going to be examining me repeatedly and prodding and peeking. Not like last time. This is not a spectator sport. When I went to the bathroom last time a bunch of that stuff dripped on my foot, Can't you just dip your swab in THAT?!"

She looked at me like I was nuts. I was soooo not nuts.

"No, it has to be a vaginal specimen."

"Well, I am no expert but it seems to me that amniotic fluid could only come from one place, and if you guys clean up around here the way you are supposed to, and seeing as I am the only patient in this unit at this time, this bodily fluid on my foot right here would have to belong to MY womb. Right?"

Eventually, I gave in. I had another mini-gush and rang the nurse to do her swab.

The conclusion was that it was indeed amniotic fluid. The question once again was when had my water broken? I was not biting.

"I believe I told you 6 p.m. That is the story I am sticking to. Now, let's get something straight. I was in here six years ago for the birth of my daughter. She was my first and I didn't know what the hell was going on, but things have changed. I don't want ANYBODY looking at my privates. The doctor gets one free exam, after that it is $5 a peek. This goes for you nurses as well. There is absolutely NO REASON for you people to be looking at my goods every 20 minutes. You put me through that last time around and it felt like 27 hours of rape. Now, where is the bag with my baked potato and chili?"

They went away and I began eating as much as I could. I was having no labor at all, just that messy little gush every once in a while. The baby was quiet, resting up for the long haul I guess. I had plowed through my baked potato and was working on my chili, the iced tea was holding up famously, when the nurse poked her head in. I could tell by the calculated look in her eye she was coveting my snack. Not one to hold punches, I laid it out on the table. "Don't think you are taking my food away. I have a marathon to run tonight and I need my oats." She merely nodded and left. I should have known better than to think that was the end of it.

Feeling restless I got up and wandered down the hall. It was 12:30 a.m., and quiet. I was alone in the panting, grunting, cussing area of the baby ward. I waddled down the hall and wondered why they strip you to your bare bum, take your clothes, and leave you with 2 meters of broadcloth to cover yourself and catch all that messy amniotic fluid that periodically leaks out your chute. I realized at that moment this entire business was designed to prevent pregnant ladies from leaving (most likely they would be on their way to the nearest fridge if they did leave). Emotions can run wild during labor and almost anything can happen but they can make sure it all happens in that ward by stealing your clothes and leaving you with a half sheet and your bum sticking out. And, believe me, 9 months gestation takes the BROAD out of broadcloth and makes that old open-backed gown look like a tea towel.

It felt good to walk. I was starting to feel some labor twinges, but the walking just felt so good! At least it felt good until I returned to my room for another go at my doggy bag only to discover it had mysteriously disappeared. HOW was I going to crap on the nurses if I didn't have a full stomach? The lonely cup of iced tea beckoned me. I wanted to take it with me but I need one hand to hold the back of my gown and the other to catch my leaking amniotic fluid. Oh, yes, they saw me coming. These nurses, they are sneaky!

I walked until 3:30 a.m., and by then I was so tired I had to stop for fear of falling asleep in mid-stride. I went from walking to sitting for what seemed like hours.

The entire time, I felt like each nurse or aide or doctor I came in contact with was merely waiting for me to say, "Okay, I was just funning you about the natural childbirth. Like, what was I thinking!?! Let's get this baby out, Start cutting!" They would look in and let me know they were right there...scalpel sharpened, hands washed...waiting...I did not budge. Every half hour or so someone would come in and say, "Are you SURE your water broke at 6 p.m.? You know the doctor is not going to let you go past 24 hours of labor." I would nod and reassure them that it was indeed 6 p.m....the countdown was on.

Fate rewarded my determination and confidence in my body. I was the only woman to appear in the labor ward that night. In fact, I was the only woman delivering a baby the next day. Not one other pregnant lady walked through those doors until I finished my job. In addition to that, I was gifted with possibly the most wonderful labor nurse in the free world. She had no other patients and she was with me from 7 a.m. until that baby presented himself to the world. I had made it quite clear that the only people I wanted in that room were the ones actively involved in the labor...and if you can't push for me, and you can't get me a cup of tea, then why are you there, really?! I even told the baby's father he was not invited. I'm sure they thought I was nuts...I am also sure there were a few who wished they had had the nerve to be just like me.

Being the only one there, no family friends or relatives, just the nurse and me, I guess that connected us in a way that she doesn't often experience.

I had my very own nurse. She was such a wonderful person. She was there every minute. She left my side every so often to step behind the curtain. She told me the next day it was to sip tea. She said it was Tim Horton's® and she didn't have the heart to drink it in front of me. Looking back, I think she was afraid to show it to me. I may have been in pain and on my back cussing and panting, but I have a farmer's reach and I would have rung her skinny neck if she had dared pull out a Tim's with no intention of sharing.

I had told my nurse at the beginning that I was not interested in a needle in my spine, not now - not ever, so don't even THINK of asking, and you know what? She never did! It only occurred to me a few days later that nobody asked me or suggested to me that a needle in my back might lessen the pain. My reasoning was that I had heard that an epidural would slow labor right down, sometimes it even halted it altogether, and I wanted my baby born "on time."

I also have to say that I went through the entire process of labor and delivery with only two vaginal exams. One when I first arrived at the hospital (that was the attending doc's freebie), and the second exam was when I finally buckled and asked my angel nurse for just a small dose of Demerol to take the edge of my pain...not enough to be happy or halt labor, but just a taste, like a swig of whiskey before they dig out the bullet. The deal was she had to examine me first to make sure I wasn't too far along, I guess. I was beyond arguing at that point.

He crowned and the doctor decided I needed help to get him out. Everything seemed to be hurried all of a sudden. He gave me the choice of forceps or vacuum extraction. I was horrified but I had to put my faith somewhere and my lungs were getting weak with the efforts. I just couldn't imagine using something that resembled a kitchen utensil on my baby's head, so I went for option B. I had no idea what that would be like, but I just said all kinds of prayers to keep my baby safe and next thing you know I pushed and his head was out. I knew it was out because, boy oh boy, can you feel that! I glanced down to see a head and what looked like a golf ball stuck under the scalp (from the extraction device) and I looked away and decided I didn't see it. "One more push!" they encouraged me. All of a sudden the doctor hollered "STOP PUSHING!!! The cord is around his neck!"

You might as well say stop sneezing, or stop falling in mid-air. Stop pushing?! As if! Well, that cord was looped twice around his neck, but the doctor

> *I was a mother and I was the boss of my birth.*

pulled it off and I pushed again and out plopped a baby. The first thing the doctor said was, "Well, will you look at this! Wow." He held up an unbelievably long umbilical cord that was tied in a big double knot half way down. He just looked at me and shook his head.

~~~~~

I took control and had my pregnancy MY way, on MY terms. I could not have imagined it turning out any better. My son was born June 12, 2005. He was born natural and weighed 7 pounds, 4 ounces.

Labor hurts. You are present for the whole thing and it hurts like nobody's business. They say you forget the pain and, well, you do, but not for a couple weeks. It was wonderful being able to carry my baby out of the hospital and to be able to do laundry and walk upright and feel good! After the c-section, it took four months before I felt normal. After a natural childbirth, they throw you a towel and point you towards the shower while they are still sucking the goo from the baby's mouth.

The entire experience (aside from having my well-planned take-out mysteriously disappear during labor) was exactly how I planned it. It was everything I had wanted from the experience, everything I could have hoped for. I had a plan. I visualized it and I had it set in my mind and we were doing things MY way this time. I was no longer a naïve, first-time mom. I was a mother and I was the boss of my birth. I had decided I would not be intimidated by anything or anyone. There were hints and comments about my health and my ability to do this, but I refused to accept these negative thoughts. At the end of the day, a mother will do what is best for her child. She will not put a baby in danger out of stubbornness. I guess it is all about recognizing and defining true risk. If you decide to go through the labor experience, you must not allow doubt into the equation. Sometimes things happen that require surgical intervention and, when it's all done, a healthy, living baby is always a wonderful outcome. However, every mother deserves unlimited support and encouragement regarding labor and childbirth. Women were designed to grow a baby and give birth and, if we are blessed to carry a child, it is because God puts His faith in us to grow and deliver and raise up a little baby. So, we need to honor that gift by doing our part!

One thing I can tell you for sure. As soon as I decided not to be a patient, that I was going to have this baby the old-fashioned way, my pregnancy became a real celebration. I felt stronger and more confident. I felt fully and most awesomely female. Pregnant, I was in my full glory. Just making that decision in my heart was so empowering! I would encourage all women to embrace this miracle we have been designed to fulfill. At the end of the day, you will do whatever you have to do to be safe and make sure your baby is safe, and sometimes that means a c-section. But it needs to be considered a safety device, not the actual appliance!

Blessings to all women!

Chaleen Duggan has been schooled in agriculture and carpentry, and is a student of natural medicine and herbology. She sees the world through a comedic filter, and enjoys making observations to a random audience. Chaleen currently resides in semi-rural Northern Ontario with her young muses, Noah and Hannah. She spends her days working on various messy projects (she can always blame the mess on the kids if company shows up). A notable work-in-progress is her ebook on Leathercrafting Projects, which will be available through Booklocker.com later this year. Chaleen can be reached at chaleenduggan@hotmail.com and will consider requests for freelance work.

4. Birth and Re-birth
by Brigid Cumming

Robert • March 5, 1992

I enjoyed myself and was enviably healthy all through my pregnancy. When I found out I was pregnant I had cut back on my smoking, finally quitting at about four months. Although heavy to begin with, I ate a good, nutritious diet and walked for exercise, which meant I gained a total of 21 pounds. I was briefly hospitalized when my blood pressure went up in my eighth month, but it came down and all was well.

One thing my husband and I didn't manage was to attend childbirth preparation classes. We did review material with our community nurse and toured the hospital delivery room and I read quite a lot on my own. My coach, Laurie, had given birth to her daughter at the local hospital. She was very enthusiastic and looked forward to supporting me during labor.

Tuesday afternoon, March 3, I started to get irregular 'twinges'. By 6 p.m. I was thinking I really should ask at my next doctor's appointment (the next day) about these painful Braxton-Hicks contractions. At 10 p.m., I began timing them and realized they were every five minutes and lasting 25-45 seconds. By 11 p.m. I decided to call my husband. He came home from work and we left for the hospital just after midnight.

It was disappointing to find out when I got to the hospital that I was only 1 cm dilated, but the nurse admitted us, and we settled into the labor room. John eventually fell asleep in the chair next to the birthing bed, but I was too excited to sleep. I ate some toast, played with the bed controls, and timed contractions. At 8 a.m. my doctor came to check on me. Not much progress to report. Shortly after, Laurie arrived, ready to coach. And, slowly, the day passed. Much to my surprise I found that visitors could appear in the labor room to 'see' me without any notice given or asked. I felt like a strange sort of zoo exhibit. The nurse put a sign on the labor room door banning visitors after I burst into tears and refused to see the fourth or fifth. It took about an hour to get me calmed down.

By mid-afternoon I was tired, discouraged and only 3 cm. I had tried massage and showers; now I asked for Demerol, which I'd never had before. It made me woozy, but dulled the pain. At 6 p.m., my doctor ruptured my membranes, hoping to speed things up. I tried Entonox gas and vomited repeatedly. More Demerol made me very sleepy, but only reduced the pain slightly. I slept between contractions, waking as they began. I could not relax, which began a downward tension/pain/fear spiral. More Demerol. B-I-G mistake. I was out of touch with my body and my surroundings, but not out of touch with the pain. An IV was put in, later removed. More Demerol. A catheter to drain my bladder. I was conscious only during the peaks of contractions... It felt like I was bobbing on an endless sea of pain. Time telescoped.

At 3 a.m. on March 5th, I woke suddenly out of a stupor. I had to push. The nurse went running for the doctor. I was checked, believed to be fully dilated, and began pushing. At 8 a.m., a second doctor was brought in to assess me. She didn't think I was fully dilated. Syntocin was begun to augment my contractions. More pushing. Attempts with the vacuum extractor failed. One nurse was in tears, both doctors were worried, and my husband, family and Laurie were exhausted and scared. I was exhausted and scared, too, but surprisingly calm. I kept asking how the baby was doing. He was fine. I hurt. I groaned my way through each contraction. My lower back was so sore it actually felt like it was on fire. I wanted this over.

Mid-morning the decision was made; nothing more could be done at that hospital. Everyone frantically made arrangements for my transfer. Another local hospital was full; there was no obstetrician in another. My doctor finally contacted a former classmate at a hospital in Vancouver who agreed to take me. We had a destination. My husband could go with me on the medevac jet; there was room. My doctor apologized for not coming, too.

I was bundled up for the trip to the airport... by fire truck? The ambulance was already in Sandspit, so surrounded by the smell of gumboots, the medevac attendant and I were off to the helipad. We flew to Sandspit, transferred to the jet, then headed for Vancouver.

I had been given a shot of Demerol just before leaving the hospital. Perhaps it relaxed me enough for my labor to finally kick in, who knows? At any rate, I was on the jet, wrapped and strapped into a stretcher, legs together and I absolutely had to push. My contractions zoomed up to 90 seconds long, every three minutes. There was nothing anyone could do. The attendant rubbed my back as I lay on my side, moaning and concentrating on not pushing.

Flying time to Vancouver took one hour. Then I was loaded onto an ambulance and we set off for the hospital, arriving there about 3:30 p.m. I had passed from moaning and writhing with each contraction to pleading for someone—anyone—to do something for the pain. I was wheeled through long narrow hallways and into an elevator heading up to maternity. John was diverted to go and fill out forms while a half-dozen people descended on me, measuring, probing, assessing. Someone waved a blank general consent form and demanded my signature. I protested weakly, but was told I must sign to get an epidural. I signed. An internal fetal monitor lead was slapped on and removed twenty minutes later. "Well—he's fine," announced the nurse. The anesthetist arrived to put in an epidural.

It took effect midway through a contraction and the complete absence of sensation was blissful. Everyone left. The obstetrician came in and briskly examined me. I asked if the delivery was going to be by forceps. "No, cesarean," she said. No discussion, no explanation, just a bald statement. I finally said, "Oh...okay." I had not expected this, but mistakenly assumed that because I'd signed a general consent form I now had no choice in the matter. It was a relief to know that things would soon be over. The obstetrician left.

John appeared while I was being prepped. His mum and sister were also at the hospital. They had raced there after being told about the medevac, as at first nobody knew if John could accompany me. I was wheeled into the operating theatre while John was sent off to change. The anesthetist put a second IV in when I told her the one I already had in was a 22. (When it had been installed, at the first hospital, the nurse had commented that it was only a 22, which is a small-size IV.) Both my arms were strapped down "just like Christ on the cross," said the anesthetist cheerily, adding "not that we're going to crucify you." I was draped and scrubbed. Nobody looked at me or explained what they were doing or why, and I was very glad when my husband came to sit beside me. I was scared.

The operation—birth?—was surprisingly quick. I could not see anything, but felt the oddest sensation as Robert was removed. The image that formed in my mind was of rummaging through a purse for something, but it was the obstetrician rummaging through me. Suddenly there was a baby in the room. For a fuzzy second, I actually wondered where he had come from. A boy, large, well-formed, crying. It was 5:33 p.m., Thursday, March 5, 1992. The nurse passed him from the obstetrician to the pediatrician. Robert was processed: weighed (9 lbs., 8.5

oz.), measured (22 inches long, 14-inch head), tested, mucus removed. My husband was congratulated and given the baby to hold. Someone reminded him to show Robert to me. John gingerly moved over to me, blocked by the now-vacant stool at my head, and I glimpsed Robert. I was mildly pleased, slightly surprised that I didn't feel much of anything except tired. After a few moments, Robert, the pediatrician, two nurses and John left. I heard a surprised voice say "Boy, she sure is bleeding a lot." And, then I fell into oblivion.

I woke up still in the operating theatre, drape still up, arms tied down, apparently unattended. There were two or three nurses putting equipment away on the other side of the room. I could hear them talking but could not see them. They finished and left. I was alone and utterly helpless. I was wondering whether I could scream loudly enough to be heard outside the operating theatre when the anesthetist bustled back in with an orderly and transferred me to recovery. Interestingly, my skin went numb all over before I began to be able to move my lower body. "I must have put too much morphine in the epidural," suggested the anesthetist before she left. She had stayed past the end of her shift to 'do' me.

I watched my blood pressure and heartbeat readings upside-down on the monitor over my head and learned how to wheedle ice chips from the nurses to sooth my gummy, dry mouth. Robert was brought out of the nursery for me to see briefly as I was transferred to my room. John and his mum came in to see how I was doing and we chatted briefly before I fell deeply asleep.

The next morning at 8:30 a.m., Robert was brought to me and I held him for the first time. The full rooming-in (hospital policy, rigorously enforced) was difficult. I felt like my insides were going to fall out whenever I moved, Robert cried a lot and I was all alone in my brand-new room on the equally brand-new maternity floor. Nurses rushed in and out, few having time to talk, although they seemed pleasant. I was up and about quickly and John came in and spent hours with us every day. Flowers came from friends and my family on the Charlottes, and we had a few visitors.

On March 10th, John and I flew home from Vancouver with Robert. "Well, you certainly have a beautiful baby," was the universal comment. Breastfeeding went well once we got past the initial awkwardness and, physically, I recovered quickly. But the details of the whole experience seemed burned on my brain and I would find myself 'there', going through it again. I felt miserable and cried several times a day for weeks. In June, I saw a counselor and was told I was experiencing post-traumatic stress and maybe postpartum depression.

This was a very difficult time, but it did pass. I went into counseling and received a lot of support from family, friends and health professionals. I read a great deal about caesareans and about Vaginal Birth after Caesarean (VBAC), and worked through some thorny emotional issues. My first experience of giving birth wasn't what I'd hoped or expected, but my healthy baby boy was the wonderful result. I think I've grown and changed in some interesting ways because of that experience; it's part of me now.

Elizabeth • November 8, 1993
John and I decided to have another child. Instead of the leisurely five or six months of (ahem) 'trying' we had anticipated, I was pregnant before Robert was a year old. Although I was delighted, I was also scared. The obstetrician (who had told me that I had a 60% to 70% chance of a vaginal delivery 'next time') had put 'severe CPD' on her operative report. I was told that usually with this diagnosis a repeat Caesarean was recommended, but the local doctors didn't object to seeking a trial of labor. I was referred to the visiting

> *I alternated between dreading having another 'too big' baby and feeling that learned medical opinion wasn't worth a pitcher of warm spit.*

obstetrician. He agreed to a trial of labor at Grace, although he only gave me a 40% chance of a vaginal delivery.

As John and I began serious planning for this birth, I realized that I didn't want and couldn't afford to sit in Vancouver for a month waiting to go into labor. I started looking for a doctor in the Nanaimo area as John's parents were in Lantzville and staying with them for the birth seemed the best option. I had already decided I wanted professional labor support this time, and discussed this with the local public health nurse. She called her counterpart in Nanaimo for suggestions and was referred to Birth Options for Nanaimo and District (BOND)[7], a consumer group dedicated to improving health care for childbearing women and their families. That was the beginning of many lengthy phone calls! I was amazed at the warmth and support I received. Everyone was so nice, so concerned and full of helpful suggestions—WOW! I began to feel a small tingle of hope somewhere under all the mounds of doubt.

In July, I found a general practitioner, Dr. Chris Fritsch[8], with privileges at the Duncan hospital. I had thoroughly researched my options, but the 'deciding factors' were whimsical. The maternity ward was peaceful and sunny the day I saw it, and all the women I talked to who had gone there not only liked it, but had very short labors. Dr. Fritsch was very gentle and

---

[7] *BOND dissolved in 1996, but former members continue to be active promoting birth choices, alternatives and supporting family-centered maternity care.*
[8] *Queen Charlotte and Masset residents may remember Dr. Fritsch, who practiced here from the early 70's until the mid-80's.*

understanding and I liked Monkeytree Clinic. The name gave me a good feeling.

By September, thanks to two early births, I had a labor support person: Dana Featherstonhaugh, a nurse and midwife, who had spent hours on the phone with me since June. She was great, unfailingly calm and confident through all my ups and downs. Dana *believed* I was going to do this. I didn't know what I believed. I had read everything, reviewed everything, picked apart, analyzed, measured and evaluated Robert's birth. I alternated between dreading having another 'too big' baby and feeling that learned medical opinion wasn't worth a pitcher of warm spit.

The last few weeks were even more manic than I had dreamed. Elizabeth 'settled' (no, not dropped—she didn't engage) on September 23rd. Robert had done this a week before I went into labor. If I followed the same pattern, I'd be giving birth on the ferry south... *panic attack!* I abruptly realized how little control I had over what was going on. I made contingency plans, and finally just hoped that nothing would happen.

Nothing happened up to and past what I figured was my due date, October 29th. The bump sagged lower and lower externally. I drank gallons of raspberry-leaf tea, 'cheered on' each Braxton-Hicks contraction, walked and waited. By November 3^{rd,} I felt desperate. We had reservations for the ferry out of Port Hardy on November 13th, my husband had to be back at work by November 15th. Dr. Fritsch set up a non-stress test and ultrasound at the hospital for Friday afternoon, November 5th. After the tests, John and I both agreed that the baby looked content to stay put so I resigned myself to waiting it out.

Saturday at noon, I was delighted to feel a particularly good twinge from my cervix, but nothing more happened. Sunday, I suddenly couldn't stand waiting. Early that afternoon, I dosed myself with castor oil[9] (yuck!), hoping this would stimulate things. I ate dinner at 6 p.m. then spent from 6:30 to 9:30 in and out of the bathroom. I wondered whether the irregular contractions I was having were strong Braxton-Hicks or mild labor and irritably decided that I was tired and going to bed. If it was labor, it would just have to wake me up.

At 11:30 p.m., my husband came to bed and I jolted awake. "That was a contraction," I realized five minutes later when the second one hit. The next came 3 minutes later, then I was having strong contractions (45-60 seconds) every 5 minutes, with small ones (30 seconds) roughly halfway between them. Then the small ones got stronger.

I was so relieved to be in labor that the first few contractions felt wonderful. After 40 minutes, I was barely coping. I focused totally on making myself feel as comfortable as possible by breathing slowly and deeply, relaxing, and moving to find good positions. My labor was intense, incredible, almost unbearably powerful. It scared me. I insisted that we call Dana NOW. John called. A contraction hit and I heard him say, "I don't think you can talk to her right now—she's got her head buried in the couch." Once it finished, I did get to the phone. I don't remember what I said but, much to my relief, she agreed to come straight away and arrived shortly before 1 a.m.

I was in the bedroom getting dressed. Dana came in, hugged me, asked how I was doing and where I thought I was. I reduced my estimate (6-7 cm) to a more plausible 4-5 cm. Dana checked and said I was about 6-7 cm, but it was hard to tell because the forewaters were bulging so far down into the birth canal. I couldn't believe it! Dana was pleased but also quite concerned that I was so far along and asked how I felt

---

[9] *Castor oil should only be taken under your healthcare provider's direction. It can be very dangerous.*

about going to the a closer hospital instead of Duncan. I felt very strongly about this—we were going to Duncan; I would simply not have the baby until we got there. We got ready to leave at once.

John drove and Dana did coaching and neck/shoulder massage from the back seat. It was warm and dark in the car and I slept between contractions. They had slowed down to every three minutes or so, but were still strong. I remember wishing I could skip every other one to get a six-minute rest. I braced my feet under the dashboard and tensed my legs, pushing the seat back alarmingly when one hit. Dana was right behind me, so got the full effect. I opened my mouth and wiggled my tongue, imagining balancing something on the tip. I made a variety of noises. At one point, I heard Dana say in a small, surprised voice, "Brigid, are you biting your seatbelt?" Yes, I was. I had just turned my head and clamped on! About halfway to Duncan, I began feeling an urge to push. I didn't bother mentioning this as my waters hadn't burst, and tried to ignore it as much as possible.

It was a shock to go from the snug, dark car to the brightly-lit hospital. As I lumbered into the emergency department, blinking like an owl, I heard a nurse call out, "Well—she's certainly in labor!" This grated; I almost turned around and walked out, but went and hid in the nearest washroom to have my next contraction instead. I refused an offer of a wheelchair and we made our way up to maternity.

We were shown straight into the birthing room. It was 3 a.m. Much to my surprise, I had already met both nurses. One had set up Friday's non-stress test and the other had given me a tour of the ward in July. Georgie ushered me into the room, got out her clipboard and pen, and began asking me questions: how long had I been in labor, when had I eaten last, what were the contractions like... I had to think, I didn't want to think, I didn't want to talk. The questions seemed like bloody stupid things to be asking. I wanted to have a shower but I had to be examined first. I WAS 9 CM! The nurse ran to phone Dr. Fritsch. The baby was fine and I was so far along they didn't bother with the 'routine' fetal monitor strip—hooray!

I asked if I could have my shower now. The nurse felt I should wait until after the doctor had examined me, but Dana suggested that I could go in until he arrived if it would make me feel comfortable. The shower was warm and dark—cave-like. I squatted down and relaxed. Dana sat nearby and we talked. The technician came and drew off blood for tests right in the shower, which was very nice. It wasn't long before Dr. Fritsch was there. I didn't want to get out of the shower. I heard Dana asking if I could be examined in the shower, but he was quite emphatic that I was to come out now. I dried off and climbed back into my two hospital gowns, one on back-to front. Dana had remembered me saying I hated having my back uncovered and had asked for an extra gown to layer on top.

It was 3:40 a.m. and I was 9+ cm dilated with my membranes bulging. But, the baby's head was still quite high, about -1. I remember the doctor looking up—he was beaming—then asking for the amnio hook. I would have protested, but he looked so pleased I didn't bother. Besides, an artificial rupture of the membranes (ARM) at 9+ cm is a bit different from one at barely 4 cm. At 4 a.m. he checked me again. My cervix had an anterior lip. I groaned—this had happened last time... He calmly reached in and held the cervix back during the next contraction. This felt like being pinched, but worked—no more anterior lip! By now it was obvious that I was wanting to push. John and Dana stationed themselves on either side of me and urged me to not push, don't push, pant, come on now... I tried to fight it, but ended up pushing anyway. I wanted Dr. Fritsch to have another look, but he had stepped out of the room. "Where is that a**hole doctor?" I demanded... Fortunately, he later said he didn't hear me.

At 4:20 a.m., another quick check. "You can push now, the baby's at +2."

I was at +2! I grinned—I was delighted—I didn't believe it. "Are you sure?" I asked. Dr. Fritsch did a mild double-take. He was quite sure. "The baby's head isn't molded to a point or anything... it's really that far down?" I was assured that the baby's head was round and, yes, it really was that far down. I began pushing.

This was the hardest part of the labor for me. I didn't feel the baby's head moving down, which I had assumed I would. Each contraction literally knocked the breath out of me and there would be this overpowering urge to bear down. I made the most amazing grunting noises! But, just as I would seem to be getting somewhere with this, I would hear Dana and John insisting that I breathe in now. By the time I had managed to gulp in air, the contraction would be gone. I soon felt totally frustrated—I only seemed to be doing this for 20-30 seconds every four to five minutes and I was having to waste half the contraction trying to suck air into my lungs. Not only that, when I complained that the contractions were tapering off and weren't strong enough, everyone seemed to think it was funny.[10]

I asked how far things had progressed. Dr. Fritsch obligingly checked and said the head was down further. "How far?" I demanded. Maybe half a centimeter. Was that all? Well, maybe it was 7 millimeters... I thought that was an improvement, then realized everyone was smiling. I was immediately suspicious. "Are you sure?" The next day I 'got' the joke, but at the time I was positively grim.

---

[10] *I saw my chart two days later and found out that my contractions had been 60 seconds long and coming every two minutes.*

I had been kneeling, hanging off the labor bar and was getting tired so Dana got me moving around on the bed. She had suggested going back in the shower to help me relax, but I rejected that out of hand. We tried squatting. My left leg cramped up. I lay on my side for about a split-second before remembering that this had been an excruciatingly painful position when I'd tried it while in labor with Robert. It was still excruciatingly painful. I semi-reclined on my back, feet braced against the bar. I found it difficult to coordinate my pushing. Dana gave me instructions and I couldn't manage to follow them—pulling up with my arms while bearing down seemed like trying to rub my stomach while patting my head. I found it impossible to think and was irritable beyond belief.

Dana and John encouraged me, massaged me and offered me sips of cold water. They were 'in touch' almost continuously—it felt so good! Only once did I feel even briefly alone and, when I quavered out, "please, somebody touch me", someone was right there. They also tried to get me to see that I was making progress. John kept encouraging me to look in the mirror, but I couldn't keep my eyes open during contractions.

Dana suggested that I feel the top of the baby's head. I didn't want to at first, but changed my mind. I couldn't tell how far down it was but it felt warm and wet, soft and wrinkled... altogether marvelous! I was amazed, but still convinced that nothing was happening, that the baby was stuck, that things were going wrong. I blurted out something of this and was both relieved and surprised when Dr. Fritsch (sounding rather puzzled) said, "But you're not doing anything abnormal."

Abruptly, everything became too much for me and I decided I wanted an epidural. I switched to all fours, face buried in the bed. This position was actually very efficient, the contractions were completely horrible. I had quite an argument going with Dana, which the nurses and Dr. Fritsch seemed not to notice at all. This came to a head as Dana was patiently saying, "Now, Brigid, remember you didn't want to use drugs" and trying to suggest some less drastic alternatives.

I yelled, "F*** philosophy, Dana! I WANT AN EPIDURAL!" and buried my head in the pillow, wailing, "Why isn't anyone listening to me? What do I have to do?"

I hadn't really been aware of anyone other than John and Dana for some time. The nurses attended to things very quietly and Dr. Fritsch puttered about in the background checking equipment, looking out the window, and then wandering back to the foot of the bed. Now, he stepped in and suggested a pudendal block and setting up the vacuum extractor. This sounded fine, but first I had to have an IV put in. Two attempts failed and I became quite impatient. (Two earlier attempts to install a heparin lock had also failed.) I wanted something for the pain right now, no more delays, and announced this very pointedly. He began to put in the pudendal block. This involved four needles which hurt like an incredibly fierce pinching followed by the gross sensation of a rather large needle going... well, let's just say it took everything I had to keep my bottom glued to the bed. It took effect very quickly and was just perfect. I now felt the contractions higher up, behind my pubic bone, and they were manageable. The vacuum extractor was applied.

On the next contraction, I pushed with everything I had (managing to coordinate arms and bottom!) and surprised myself by screaming loudly through about three octaves. The nurse had arranged the mirror so I could see what was going on and I kept my eyes open—no way was I going to miss this! There was an incredible sense of pressure and movement (finally!) and Elizabeth's head emerged wearing the vacuum extractor like an off-center crazy pink pillbox hat. There was a baby coming out of me!

I was ecstatic, then I heard Dr. Fritsch say very quietly that her cord was wound around her neck. I panicked and pushed, even though I wasn't having a contraction. I abruptly realized that this might make things worse and stopped pushing.

Fortunately, her cord loosened off instead of tightening. Dr. Fritsch cut and clamped it and told me I had to get her out with the next contraction. The words were hardly out of his mouth when the next contraction began. Another incredible push and yell and out she slithered. I was looking straight at the clock and knew what time it was, but I still asked the nurse when she had been born. It was 5:45 a.m., Monday, November 8, 1993.

Dr. Fritsch laid her gently on me. I welcomed her, and then she was taken by the nurse and suctioned. A couple of minutes later I felt a mild contraction—all 'pins and needles'—and the placenta slithered out like so much warm gelatin. It was a couple of minutes more before I got to hold Elizabeth but I didn't mind. I could see and hear her and I felt wonderful. She was weighed and measured—8 lbs. 9.5 oz., 22 inches long, 13.5-inch head.

"See, I told you she was a girl," said Dr. Fritsch. (He had predicted this about three weeks earlier.) I held her, then passed her around. I had a third degree tear from delivering both shoulders simultaneously, so Dr. Fritsch spent about an hour stitching me up. Dana made me three cups of tea and gave me a fruit cup (I had brought supplies with me), as I was suddenly intensely hungry and thirsty.

We all admired Elizabeth and then the nurses went off to get ready for shift change. Shortly after that, John and Dana left for home and well-deserved sleep. Dr. Fritsch came back in at about 7:30 a.m. and we chatted for a few minutes. Then it was just me and Elizabeth for about half-an-hour. It was a gorgeous fall morning, clear, crisp and the sun just poured in the birthing room windows. Birth and re-birth; an amazing cycle.

Brigid Cumming, 41, lives with her husband John, son Robert, daughter Elizabeth and a herd of house-rabbits in Port Clements on the Queen Charlotte Islands (Haida Gwaii) off the northwest coast of British Columbia, Canada. When not gazing blearily at deer browsing in her back yard at 5:30 a.m., she can generally be found on her computer, reading a book, or at a meeting. You can e-mail her at bcumming@island.net if you would like a copy of "Islands Birth Stories", a collection of Queen Charlotte Islands birth stories.

5. A Tale of Two Sons
by Patrice Fagnant-MacArthur

My induction was planned for 6 p.m. on a Monday night. I was 42 weeks pregnant and my baby boy showed no signs of being eager to come into the world. Surprisingly, when the nurse hooked me up to a monitor, she discovered that I was actually in the early stages of labor, having mild but unproductive contractions. I was not dilated at all. By 11 p.m., it was decided that some Pitocin was needed to help move things along. With the induction, the contractions came fast and furious.

I was left to labor through the night. A nurse would check on me periodically but, for the most part, it was just me and my husband. Thank goodness for him! As my insides felt like they were being crushed to pieces, I held his hands, looked into his eyes, and struggled to remember my Lamaze breathing. All the different positions I had learned in childbirth class were useless. Strapped to two different monitors and an IV, the most I could do was move slightly onto my side. I tried to pray but could barely form the words. Nothing seemed to help the indescribable pain.

Meanwhile, my baby was experiencing distress of his own. His heart rate kept dropping below acceptable levels. The nurse hooked me up to an oxygen mask to try to help that situation, but the mask made me feel claustrophobic and I could no longer practice my breathing. To make matters worse, my baby's heartbeat wasn't improving.

> Strapped to two different monitors and an IV, the most I could do was move slightly onto my side.

At about 9 a.m., my doctor came in and checked me. I was

finally dilated to 3 cm. and able to get an epidural. While I had dreamed of a drug-free labor, after ten hours of intense pain I was exhausted and welcomed the relief. Within minutes of receiving the epidural, the baby's heartbeat dropped even further and my contractions had slowed as well. This was one labor that didn't seem to be progressing anywhere and the doctor suggested that a c-section would be the best course of action.

I was prepped and wheeled into the operating room where my arms were stretched out and strapped as if I were on a cross. Because I had already received an epidural, the anesthesiologist simply increased the level of medicine that I was receiving through that. My husband sat next to me, holding my hand, and the doctor was ready to begin.

David came into the world at 9:40 a.m. on Tuesday, April 10, 2001. It was wonderful to hear my baby boy's first cry, a high-pitched chirp that will forever be etched into my memory. One of the nurses brought little David over to me. I couldn't touch him, but I could see him. He weighed in at 8 lbs. 1 oz. and 22 inches long, with a head slightly misshapen from being wedged in my birth canal. He was a beautiful, healthy little boy!

As my doctor started to put me back together, I began to have difficulty breathing. I turned to my husband and told him, "I can't breathe!" I heard the anesthesiologist who was monitoring my vital signs tell the doctor that I was fine – everything was normal. But I was still gasping for air. I turned to the anesthesiologist. "Please help me," I begged.

I woke up in a recovery room about an hour later. My husband was sitting nearby holding David. He told me that the doctor said I had experienced a panic attack and that they had given me general anesthesia to finish the procedure. This explanation made no sense to me. Why then? David had been born and

> *They cared about both me and my unborn child. I would recommend midwife care to anyone.*

was fine. Everything was going well. If anything, I was more relaxed then as opposed to the fifteen previous hours. Regardless of the reason, however, this was not an experience I had any desire to repeat.

When I found out I was expecting our second child a mere ten months later, I was determined to have a VBAC. Our insurance had changed and going to my previous physician was no longer an option. I began to explore different healthcare providers and decided to go to a midwife practice that was connected to a standard OB/GYN office. I reasoned that would be the best of both worlds. I would have the more natural care of a midwife (which I thought would be my best chance of having a VBAC) as well as access to more advanced medical care in the event something went wrong.

I was very impressed by the prenatal care that I received from the midwives. While I never had any complaints with the care I received from my previous OB/GYN, the midwives spent so much more time with me. They cared about both me and my unborn child. I would recommend midwife care to anyone. When I told the story of my previous c-section and the experience of not being able to breathe, I was informed that was actually a fairly common side effect of having an epidural being used during a c-section. I may have had a panic attack, but it was triggered by an actual sensation. That information made me feel better about my first birth.

Together, the midwives and I decided that if it got to the point where I needed to be induced again, I would go for a planned c-section, but otherwise I would try for the VBAC. How I wanted to have a successful vaginal birth! Even if I survived another c-section, I couldn't imagine how I would cope with a 6-week recovery period caring for a 19-month-old and a new baby.

At 41 weeks, the c-section was planned for the following Monday. How I hoped that my baby would cooperate and that I would go into labor on my own. I got my wish. Saturday night, my water broke and we headed to the hospital. The midwife was amazing. She stayed with me through the whole labor. The difference between natural labor and induced labor was incredible[11]. For a long time, the contractions were actually manageable. The midwife had me up and trying different positions. She was so supportive and encouraging.

After nine hours, though, the pain was extremely intense. I had finally reached 3 cm. and could once again have an epidural. Within minutes, my baby's heartbeat started dropping quickly. The midwife did what she could to try to get the baby's heart rate up, but it was to no avail. This time there was no conversation about whether to have a c-section. It was a matter of getting the baby out as soon as possible.

Even though the midwife's job was technically done and I was now in the doctor's hands, she stayed right by my side through the entire procedure. Her support meant so much to me. Isaac made his grand entrance at 9:55 a.m. on Sunday, November 10, 2002. As the doctor lifted him out, a collective gasp went up through the room, "Look at the size of that baby!" He checked in at nine and a half pounds, 21½ inches long, and was as chubby as could be. Thankfully, I made it through the rest of the procedure without incident.

---

[11] *Many women who have experienced both natural childbirth and induced labor report that medications used for inductions can create longer, more intense, and much more painful transactions.*

> *Bonding takes place in the heart, not the birth canal.*

Even though the outcome wasn't what I hoped, I'm glad that I opted to try for the VBAC. My second time around in labor was a much more positive experience. I have come to the conclusion, however, that how you give birth to your children (or even if you don't give birth to them, as in the case of adoption) has very little to do with being a mother. Bonding takes place in the heart, not the birth canal. What makes you a mother are late-night feedings, rocking a child, kissing boo-boos, playing, laughing, and crying together. Without a c-section, the chances are good that neither one of my children would be here. I have two beautiful, healthy boys. The scar on my abdomen was an incredibly small price to pay for the gift of my children.

Patrice Fagnant-MacArthur wrote of her experience of pregnancy and the first year of motherhood in her book, <u>Letters to Mary from a Young Mother</u>. She is the editor of http://www.spiritualwoman.net and the corresponding blog http://spiritualwomanthoughts.blogspot.com as well as a columnist on Catholicmom.com.

6. Three Births, Two VBACs
by Lea Date

When my son was born in 1990, I hated the Pitocin drip that induced twelve hours of intermittent labor. I hated the IV, and I also hated the internal monitor.

I dearly loved the kind nurse who helped me stay curled up while I was given the Epidural for a c-section when labor had failed to progress. And I knew I didn't want another cesarean if I could avoid it...although I had no complications. Actually, having staples hold my belly together was kind of cool. I recovered quickly.

Two years later, different town, different hospital, different insurance, different doctor (family practice this time). Our second child arrived ten days early and was three pounds smaller. And my labor was just as uncomfortable and annoying as the induced labor had been. I still hated the internal monitor and the IV, but hadn't been able to talk my way out of having them. No problems with the process, although the doctor had to hurry to get to the hospital on time (and the nurses were afraid I'd start screaming during the prospective parent tour, which was going on at the same time. I didn't scream). I went home with a third-degree laceration followed by a brief breast infection, but a successful VBAC. And, most importantly, a new daughter.

Two more years later. Again, a different town, different hospital, different insurance, different doctor. Having moved "back home" two months before the baby was due, we went with a family recommendation this time: the doctor who had helped with our niece's birth. He listened to my history, commenting that postnatal recovery after a severe laceration was more difficult than recovery from a C-section. He said we could try labor without an internal monitor since there had been no problems two years before. So, with impeccable timing (!) we went to the hospital at 6:00 a.m. on what should have been my husband's first day at his new job.

The maternity wing was short staffed; our nurse was in the middle of her second shift of the day and was also helping with another, more complicated birth. We reveled in the neglect! Since nobody had hooked me up to a monitor yet, we walked around the wing. I wondered why anybody suggested this as a good idea for a laboring activity; once around was plenty for me. By the time we got back to the birthing room, the nurse was available to hook me up...this time to an external monitor, but still with an IV. I settled into the bed while my husband called home to let his parents know how we were doing. We listened to the cassettes we'd brought...some were the same ones we'd listened to during previous births. The doctor came in and my husband's sister (the one who'd recommended the doctor) came in and stayed. After the other birth down the hall was successfully achieved, our nurse came in. We were too occupied to change the cassette; the same one played over and over. I remember thinking that if I had to listen to it a fourth time, I'd hate it for the rest of my life.

I'd always heard what a relief the "pushing" part of labor was. Not for me...pushing took forever, and nobody had ever heard me groan so loudly. Our baby, another daughter, was born.

That time, there were no complications. Six days later I was hiking (slowly) with extended family, including my visiting mother, in a nearby redwood forest.

Over the years, Lea Date has told the story of her children's births many times, usually for the sake of embarrassing them.

7. Three VBACs!
by Carrie Steinweg

My first son was born naturally after a long, induced labor. Seeing my beautiful 7 pound, 3½ ounce little bundle instantly made it all worthwhile. However, it must have been rougher than I now recall, because it was five years before our next son was born.

Our second little guy arrived three weeks early at six pounds, five ounces via emergency c-section because of a complication with the placenta. When his heart rate dropped dangerously low and didn't show signs of coming back up, there was no choice but to rush me to the operating room. I think the entire procedure took about 11 minutes. I was happy to finally have him here, but had no idea what I was in for when it came to the recovery. The gas pains were unbearable and the pain medication had me so out of it that I would fall asleep in mid-sentence while my sisters were visiting me in the hospital. Once I came home, taking care of myself, my new baby and my five-year-old was no easy task. It was truly 12 full weeks before I felt like I was back to normal. I hoped I'd never have to go through a recovery like that again. And if it was that hard with two children, what would it be like when there were three?

Luckily, when I became pregnant with my third son, about 20 months later, I went back to see the obstetrician who had delivered my first 2 children and learned that her daughter had joined the practice. I saw the daughter for my first appointment and she was just as lovely and calm as her

> *I hoped I'd never have to go through a recovery like that again.*

mother. I expressed my wishes to have a VBAC, even though I didn't know too much about it at that point. She was very understanding and explained that the complication that occurred in my last delivery wouldn't necessarily recur this time around, so there was no reason not to attempt a VBAC. Knowing that my doctor and I were on the same page was a big relief.

Even when I developed gestational diabetes, which can result in large babies that have a hard time being delivered vaginally, my doctor still had no problem with me attempting a VBAC.

The labor went pretty smoothly and at no time was there any indication that a c-section might be needed. For some reason, the epidural I received had only taken on my right side but, other than that, everything went perfect. My sister-in-law, who was a registered nurse in the newborn nursery, happened to be working that day and was in the room for the delivery. It had been my easiest labor and delivery so far and he was the first of my kids that was completely healthy and came home on time (my first spent 10 days in neo-natal for a lung infection and the second spent his first few days in special care for an extreme case of jaundice, followed by a return to the emergency room two days later that resulted in a three-day stay in the pediatric unit, again for jaundice.) He was a healthy 7 pounds, 10 ounces with a full head of red hair.

Once I was home, my recovery was so easy compared to the weeks following my c-section. Like most new moms, I jumped into doing a little too much too soon. Within a week, I was driving, carrying my toddler around, and going up and down stairs easily. It felt wonderful to be able to do so many things for myself.

With the exception of some difficulty with nursing during the first month, the six-week recovery period was wonderful. Had I had another c-section, I really don't know how I would have handled it. My mom had come over to cook some meals and help with the kids after my c-section. This time her health prevented her from being there. My husband was working two jobs and even though I'd requested a one-year maternity leave, like I'd taken with my two previous pregnancies, my bosses insisted that I return at the 12-week mark. Had I been returning that soon after having a c-section, I know I would have been a mess.

A year after the arrival of son number three, we found out that another baby was on the way. Since I'd had a successful VBAC already, I was confident that I could do it again. I had the same doctor through my pregnancy that had been there for my VBAC and she was fully supportive again, despite another diagnosis of gestational diabetes. I spent a pretty short time in the hospital during my labor – about six hours before the delivery. My doctor's mom (who had delivered my first two) was down the hall for another delivery and made it into the room just as the nurse checked and called out, "Hurry up, get the doctor in here!" This little guy wasn't so little. At 8 pounds, 5 ounces, he was quite a butterball, but the labor and delivery was easier than the last one.

Fast forward another 12 months and we are somewhat surprised to learn that we'll be having our fifth child. A few months after returning from maternity leave after my third one was born, I quit my full-time job of 12 years to work at home and be with my children around the clock. Changes in insurance had caused us to opt for a less expensive HMO coverage that would cover immunizations and well check ups for our growing family. We were happy with it so far, but I was heartbroken to have to look for a new obstetrician, since the mother and daughter duo that had delivered my four boys were not in our insurance plan.

At the suggestion of my sister-in-law, I went to a doctor affiliated with the same hospital. The doctor was a male who was very friendly and experienced, but was hesitant about doing VBAC's. At each visit, he'd remind of the risks. Then I'd remind him that I had delivered two babies by VBAC already without complications. When I did go for the extended glucose tolerance test and it came back high, he explained the likelihood of this baby being even bigger than the last and perhaps making a VBAC complicated. He listened to my concerns, but in the back of my head, I kept wondering if I'd get to the delivery room and he'd chicken out and do surgery.

During the pregnancy, I followed my dietary guidelines carefully so that I wouldn't gain more than the recommended 25 pounds and would decrease the chances of having a huge newborn. I gained a total of 24 pounds.

My fifth labor went very quickly once I got to the hospital. About four hours after my arrival, our fifth son was born, weighing 8 pounds, 2 ounces. It turned out that we went to the hospital on a Friday night and our son didn't arrive until 2:13 a.m., so another doctor was on call for Saturday. It was a doctor I'd never met. There was no discussion about c-section. By the time the doctor got in the room, I was fully dilated and ready to go. All my fretting had come to an end and I was soon the mom of five who'd experienced a natural delivery, a c-section and three successful VBAC's.

Carrie Steinweg is a freelance writer who resides in Chicago's south suburbs with her husband and five sons. She has written for over 20 publications, including Chicago Baby, Chicago Parent, Springfield Parent, Healthy Family, Fire Rescue, 9-1-1 *and* Auto and RV. *She is a correspondent for the Times Newspapers of Northwest Indiana and also writes a parenting column for that publication. She is the author of two pictorial* history books by Arcadia Publishing, *Images of America: Lansing, Illinois* and *Images of America: South Holland, Illinois.*

8. A Belly Dancer's VBAC
by Heidi Wessman Kneale

It took me five years to fall pregnant with my first daughter. While the pregnancy was no fun, I did look forward to giving birth and holding the child I'd been yearning for after so many years. I did my research and came up with an impressive birth plan that covered *everything*, including the need for a cesarean.

When my due date came and went and was soon a distant memory, and I still hadn't gone into labor, my obstetrician scheduled me for an induction. I had regular but faint contractions. By 12 hours, I'd only dilated a few centimeters. Since my baby was in no distress and I was fine, they broke my waters and sat back to wait.

It was a very long wait. Everything was fine, but 36 hours was a long time to wait! "I'm sorry," my obstetrician told me. "We'll have to perform a cesarean."

"No!" I wailed. He knew how much I wanted to deliver naturally. But I had only dilated nine centimeters. "Here's the deal," he said. "We'll take you down and prep you for surgery. If you are fully dilated to 10, I'll attempt a forceps delivery."

Fear can accomplish many things. It was only half an hour from announcement to laying me out on the operating table, but when my obstetrician discovered that I was the requisite ten centimeters and fully effaced, he was true to his word; he went in with the "salad spoons". He secured my baby's head and got her turned, but couldn't get her to descend properly. "I'm sorry, but I don't want her head to pop off like a daisy. We'll have to perform a cesarean."

For several days, I had more tubes coming out of me than the London Underground.

As the green curtain went up, I reminded him of my birth plan. "Be sure to use the kind of incision that allows for VBAC." I had requested a low-transverse uterine incision, or "bikini" incision, the type best suited for VBACs. This incision allows muscle tissue to knit a scar that is much stronger than the older types of incisions.

My daughter, Sarah, was born safe and sound, I got what my obstetrician called a "Happy Face Scar" and I was wheeled up to the maternity ward to rest and recover, assured that my daughter was well and that my "liver and kidneys look nice and healthy." Good to know, I guess, but I never thought I'd ever have anyone looking at me from the inside while I was still living.

For several days, I had more tubes coming out of me than the London Underground. Once I was unassimilated, I went down for X-rays. My obstetrician wanted to know why my daughter wouldn't properly descend. The result: my pelvis measured fine, but for one measurement. "Borderline," my obstetrician told me. "You might be able to give birth vaginally next time, but only if the baby is small enough." Otherwise, he considered me an excellent candidate for a VBAC.

All other indicators also favored a natural subsequent delivery. I had had a healthy, progressive labor and uncomplicated recovery. I was in excellent general health, being a belly dancer.

Six months later, my dear husband and I neglected the birth control. Much to our surprise, I was pregnant again! "You know I want a VBAC," I told my obstetrician.

"Well, that all depends on the baby, doesn't it?" He was willing to let me try for a VBAC, but only under certain conditions: I had to go into labor naturally, I had to progress, and I was not allowed any form of pain relief other than nitrous oxide (called "laughing gas" or "gas and air").

His biggest concern was uterine rupture. While the risk of one is generally less than 2%[12], a uterine rupture is serious business. It means a cesarean for sure, possible hysterectomy, and even potential death of the mother and/or baby. No wonder my obstetrician had concerns.

But I'd been through a caesarian and I swore that, if it was in my power, I would have a VBAC.

So I did more research. What would induce labor? Massage, acupuncture, raspberry leaf tea, herbal mixtures featuring dong quai and both cohoshes (black cohosh and blue cohosh), falling from great heights, castor oil...

I struck the last two from my list. There was no way I was taking castor oil. Ick! And my midwife discouraged its use because too much could cause a laxative effect in the baby, and swallowing meconium was not a nice start to life. I wasn't too keen on the falling thing, either. However, there was a rather large water slide at the local pool...

---

[12] *Statistics vary depending on where you look, but some believe the chance of uterine rupture during a VBAC with a prior lower transverse scar and the strict avoidance of labor inducing/augmenting drugs puts the risk at only one-half percent (.5%). Some studies suggest an even lower percentage. See: http://www.home birth.org.uk/vbacsigns.htm*

The massage worked well, in getting my baby to drop, but within an hour of moving around, she rose right back up again. Acupuncture, same thing. I'd been taking the herbs under the care of a naturopath for over a month, and had no idea if they were working or not. I'd had no changes in my Braxton-Hicks, nor any indication that I would go into labor soon.

My obstetrician scheduled my cesarean on a Tuesday, the day after I was due. One week before that, I got desperate. I had hoped to go into an earlier labor, for a smaller baby would have a better chance of fitting through. An ultrasound on the Wednesday before confirmed a small head. "She looks lovely," the ultrasound doctor told me. "She'll fit through just fine."

Hallelujah! Now, if only I could get labor going.

Consulting my list, I discovered I'd tried everything except the falling and the castor oil.

Falling it was. On Thursday, I took myself down to the local pool and went down their giant water slide four times. I would have gone down a fifth, but those three flights of steps were getting tougher and tougher to climb.

Friday morning, I got what I thought were Braxton-Hicks. Since they came and went, like in the past, I didn't pay much attention to them. Then towards the evening, they grew stronger. These were no Braxton-Hicks, this was full labor.

My husband had gone to a computer gaming night, with my blessing, as this probably would be the last time for the next few months he'd be able to. This was before I realized I was in labor. Once I'd confirmed I was in labor, I called the hospital and let them know I was a VBAC candidate.

Normally, the midwives prefer that a laboring woman remain at home until her contractions get to a certain point. But, they wanted me to come in immediately. I called my dear husband and he took me to the hospital.

I was hooked up to a machine that went 'bing!' and given a button to push. I had to push the button every time the baby moved. No problem there, but my finger did get tired during the twenty minutes she had hiccups.

Things progressed nicely. I dilated a centimeter an hour and looked like I would give birth some time on Saturday morning.

This concerned my midwives and obstetrician. While he had no problems with my attempting a VBAC, he was still a cautious man, for this particular Saturday morning the whole surgical wing had been shut down. The hospital was going through some much-needed upgrades and chose Saturday, with no scheduled surgeries, to turn off the water supply.

"We'll have to send you to the private hospital," he told me.

"But I can't afford a private hospital!"

He reassured me. "This hospital has an agreement with the private hospital," which was only a three-minute drive away, "to take any emergency surgical cases. You won't be charged."

I didn't need any more convincing.

What a change from the public hospital! Unlike the overcrowded maternity ward there (as it was a full moon that weekend), there was nobody but me at the private hospital. I received the full attention of the midwives where they kindly assured me that, yes, I could have the chicken tortellini in a cream sauce followed by Black Forest cake after I gave birth as

I was still a cesarean candidate, but would I like a complimentary newspaper to read between contractions instead? Meanwhile, I entertained them with belly rolls and figure-eights from belly dancing. After the first midwife got over her initial shock (I shocked a midwife!) she called all the others in to watch. "You should have no problems giving birth," they said, watching my stomach ripple.

I even got my choice of a birthing room. "Would you like purple, the green or the blue?" I chose green and was given as much nitrous oxide as I could suck through the happy pipe.

By this point, I had dilated to ten centimeters and, as far as my obstetrician could tell, there was no sign of a potential uterine rupture, and the baby's vital signs were fine. Her head was engaging properly in my pelvis, thanks to the figure-eights.

Then came the second stage of labor. I never reached second stage with my first baby, so this was a new experience. If uterine rupture were going to happen, it would happen now, when the contractions were at their strongest.

So what did the midwives do? They took away my happy pipe! I had to be alert to the signals of my own body so I could notify the obstetrician if anything went wrong.

Everything went fine. My time drew near and I crowned. I needed a minor episiotomy and ventouse (vacuum) extraction, but my beautiful girl, Amy, was born naturally. I'd had my wish and delivered a subsequent child via VBAC.

And I enjoyed my Black Forest cake.

Heidi Wessman Kneale is an Australian writer of moderate repute. By day, she works computer miracles for the local library. The rest of the time she writes books and raises babies.

9. Trading Fear for Love
by Julia Duncan

My son's birth by cesarean section is among the worst birth stories I've ever heard. Following induction at four weeks postdates, I labored for seven hours on Pitocin and was diagnosed with "failure to progress" and mild fetal distress. My son was fine, though two and a half weeks post term, but I developed a stubborn infection of unknown source and was in the hospital for ten days total. The doctors were concerned that my immune system would shut down under the effects of increasingly strong antibiotics, and one physician told my husband to prepare for the worst. My physical recovery took months; the emotional trauma stayed with me for many years. It's a story I've written down but cannot read to this day without crying in grief.

My husband and I were devotedly careful not to get pregnant again for six years. When I learned that I was expecting another child, the first thing I did was look for a direct-entry midwife who would attend a home VBAC. Against the advice of many people, I was determined not to end up on another operating table if there were any way to avoid a surgical birth.

I developed gestational diabetes at about three months and spent the next six eating on a rigid schedule and walking two miles or more almost every day. I found a wonderful, experienced midwife who believed in me, in my body, and in my baby. I enrolled in Birthworks (http://www.birthworks.org), a birthing class specific to parents planning VBAC, and studied everything I could find. My local chapter of the International Cesarean Awareness Network - ICAN (http://www.ican-online.org) served as an invaluable support group throughout the preparations.

I worried mostly about two things--that I wouldn't go into labor and that I would become exhausted, which had happened to a friend attempting a home birth. My midwife assured me again and again that I would go into spontaneous labor this time,

> *I ate and drank, went outside, meditated, visualized, danced, bathed, sang, and cried as I felt moved to, and no one interrupted me every five minutes to measure something.*

and indeed I did, on the day after my supposed "due date." Labor began on a Tuesday evening with the loss of the mucus plug and, by the next morning, I was experiencing mild contractions every ten or so minutes. They became steadily stronger, and we notified the midwife, who was on vacation at the beach some 100 miles away, so she would have time to return.

She arrived late Wednesday afternoon, at which point labor was going as expected. The contractions were still eight or so minutes apart, but getting ever stronger. My doula came over and we made sure everything was prepared. The experience of labor couldn't have been more different from the first time. I was in my own home, with my family and friends around me. I ate and drank, went outside, meditated, visualized, danced, bathed, sang, and cried as I felt moved to, and no one interrupted me every five minutes to measure something. The people with me had faith in the process instead of in machines and charts.

My body was doing its job this time. Unfortunately, Mother Nature didn't cooperate. About seven on Wednesday evening, a violent thunderstorm knocked out our electricity. That was nowhere in the plans and, needless to say, my mind rebelled ("This isn't how it's supposed to be!") and my body just quit.

Contractions subsided to fifteen or twenty minutes apart. I fell asleep, and the midwife, her aide, and my doula went home. The lights stayed out until after two in the morning, and I dozed until dawn.

Labor picked up again and, when the midwife returned, my cervix was fully effaced, but dilated to only four cm. That was as far as I got the first time and, despite trying everything from squatting to chanting to walking (and walking and walking...), I stayed at four cm all day and into the night. My three attendants stayed overnight on futons in our living room while my dear husband cooked for and took care of all of us. Labor stayed active, but I made no progress. At one point, my midwife looked me in the eye and said, "You do not have to re-experience the first labor!"

That didn't help. She theorized that my baby's head was not bearing down directly on the cervix but, again, squatting in an attempt to shift her into a more direct position didn't help. Around noon on Friday, examination showed I was still just a hair more than 4 cm dilated, and the midwife recommended we rupture the amniotic sac to get things moving. Tired by then, I agreed.

Labor immediately intensified. It became so intense, in fact, that my daughter was born 45 minutes later! I didn't even have the presence of mind to get out of bed and into the squatting position I had assumed I would give birth in. I lay on my left side with my doula holding my right leg up and out of the way-- her tears hit my daughter's head as she was born. To this day, we consider this woman my daughter's "goddess mother."

Hannah Grace was seven pounds and perfect. She didn't even cry until the following day, and I remain convinced that she was such a happy, calm baby because everyone at her birth already loved her. In the hospital with my son, the surgeon and her nurse had discussed over my sliced-open abdomen what toppings they wanted on their dinner pizza. At home with my daughter, everyone respected the sacred moment of birth.

I would go through those two and a half days of labor again without hesitation. The struggle to give birth on my own terms was worth every moment of doubt and effort. We traded the terror of my son's surgical birth for love, acceptance, and support, and the experience went a long way toward healing the bitterness and anguish of my first child's entrance into the world.

Direct-entry midwives have to be brave to practice in today's atmosphere in the U.S.A., and birthing parents have to be ready to learn as much as they can and to fight for what they know is right for their family. My midwife and all the other people who accepted and supported me in my effort to give birth naturally in my own home will always be among my greatest and most cherished heroes.

Julia Duncan is a writer and editor living in Alexandria, Virginia, with her husband, Richard Waldrop, and their children, Kai and Hannah Grace. She can be reached at stark.don@verizon.net.

10. A Natural Delivery is Best for Baby
by Diane Craver

After experiencing three vaginal deliveries with our daughters and a c-section with our son, Bart, my husband, Tom, and I definitely wanted a vaginal delivery with our fifth baby. I believed (and still do) for several reasons that having a natural delivery is usually best for the baby, the mother, and the family. Not all agree with my philosophy. A girlfriend of mine had c-sections so she wouldn't have to experience labor, and she wouldn't have to wait to see when labor would start. She loved scheduling her babies' births. I know she isn't alone in delivery preference. Since she never had a vaginal delivery, she didn't realize how different the experience is.

So, when Bart was a toddler, I was thrilled to be having another child, but concerned about avoiding a c-section. Several things ran through my mind about his birth. For one thing, cesareans aren't favorable to bonding. I had little time with him before he was taken away to a special newborn nursery. Little did I know that this would not be the only separation for our new mother/son relationship. Then, another problem occurred because our five-year-old daughter, Christina, expected to see the birth, and went to the hospital with us and my mother. Since Bart was in a breech position, a sonogram was done while I was in labor. After seeing it, my obstetrician recommended a cesarean delivery because Bart's head looked large. He said with the breech position and large head, our baby could have learning disabilities if he was delivered vaginally. But guess what? Bart's head wasn't large after all. Later, a friend of mine who is a registered nurse informed me that you can't judge size using sonograms. The heads sometimes do appear larger than they actually are.

The nurses knew Christina attended a delivery orientation class and didn't get to watch her brother being born because of the c-section. They made an exception and allowed her to hold Bart for a few minutes. I was happy to see her big smile as she held him. She had prayed for a brother and wanted one so much.

> *I didn't want any separation and wanted the baby with me as much as possible after birth. I didn't want either of us to have to recover from surgery, and I wanted to feel like a mother, not a patient, this time around.*

A really bad thing occurred after we were discharged from the hospital and back at home. I woke up during the night feeling very disoriented. When I saw my temperature, I realized why I felt confused. I was running a fever of 103 degrees. I was admitted to the hospital for a kidney infection and was a patient for a few days. Needless to say, I never had this happen after my vaginal deliveries. Fortunately, friends and relatives helped Tom take care of Bart so he could work, visit me and run errands. While Tom was gone, a church friend accidentally gave Bart regular milk instead of the prepared bottles of my breast milk. I'm happy to say that Bart survived this motherless time and is now a good-looking college man.

When I went to my first prenatal visit for our fifth child, Emily, I made sure the obstetrician and I were on the same page about me having a vaginal delivery. I didn't want any separation and wanted the baby with me as much as possible after birth. I didn't want either of us to have to recover from surgery, and I wanted to feel like a mother, not a patient, this time around. Since Sara, Christina, and April were all delivered vaginally, that was in the positive column for me. Another plus was that I had the transverse incision with Bart's cesarean so the already rare occurrence of having uterine rupture during labor was lowered even more.

I took third-grader Christina and first-grader April to the required hospital class so they could be with us during the birth. I felt the sibling bond would be deepened if they witnessed their sibling coming into the world. Christina was concerned about when the baby would be born. She wanted her own birthday and didn't know about sharing it with a younger sibling, especially a boy. Since baby Craver was due on September 15th, making it ten days ahead of Christina's, I told her that she was safe. I didn't anticipate going too much over my due date with a fifth baby. Was I ever wrong!

I went into labor at 1:00 p.m. on September 24th so was relieved I had baked Christina's birthday cake ahead and had her treats ready to pass out on her special day to her classmates. I finished doing several loads of laundry and pigged out on Little Debbie® peanut butter wafers. Hey, I knew I might need energy and probably wouldn't get anything to eat later in labor. Three-year-old Bart wasn't happy that he couldn't go with me to the hospital. He and eleven-year-old Sara, our firstborn, were going to Grandma's. Sara was born with Down syndrome and we were afraid the birth might be upsetting to her. I checked my bag and noticed I was missing several items. I knew where to look. During my pregnancy, Bart had taken my hairbrush, maternity tops, and other things of mine. I always found them under his pillow or bed.

The hospital required that an adult be with the girls in the birthing room because, in case something went wrong, they'd have to leave. And having another adult present was important to keep the children calm. I called my sister-in-law, Denise, but she wasn't sure she'd be able to leave her beauty shop in time for the event. I called another sister-in-law, Mary, at work. As it turned out, they both made it by the time I arrived at the hospital. I have to admit I hated it when the nurse had the nerve to ask me my weight right in front of them. With wide eyes, I tried to see if they were listening and whispered my weight.

While I made frequent trips to the bathroom, Denise French-braided April's hair, and the girls found orange Popsicles in the small hospital room freezer to eat. Finally, after watching *The Cosby Show*, things started getting very exciting.

I never had epidurals with our other daughters and wanted to have another drug-free delivery. Unfortunately, the pain was so bad that I started wondering if I'd made a mistake. Aunt Denise and Aunt Mary each held a girl. The aunts looked worried as they watched me dealing with the pain and intense contractions. They clutched their nieces tightly as I pushed. Both Christina and April sometimes had trouble seeing what was going on with both women sometimes blocking their views. For a few contractions, I couldn't push because of the extreme pain. Finally, the pain became so severe that I gave the biggest push ever, and the baby flew out so fast that the doctor almost didn't catch her. He was no longer puzzled about my pain since Emily's face was up instead of the usual down position[13]. He said that was why the pain was worse than usual.

We welcomed Emily Catherine into the world at 11:49 p.m. Tom teased Christina how Emily's birthday would be before hers each year. He grinned and said, "You'll get the leftover birthday cake."

Denise was certainly thankful that she was there for my VBAC, and was still on a high when she got home. My brother-in-law couldn't understand why she was so excited about seeing a baby being born since they had three children. She said, "That was different. All of our babies were delivered by c-section."

---

[13] *To read more about how a baby's position affects childbirth, see:* http://www.home birth.org.uk/ofp.htm

We were so happy that it turned out the way we wanted with having a vaginal delivery after a cesarean. April and Christina still laugh about their nervous aunts squeezing them so hard. I guess sometime before the blessed event they should have attended a class to learn how to remain calm for the children. Emily is now first in her senior class in high school, and her birth is a pleasant and remarkable family memory.

After watching the original movie, Cheaper *by the Dozen, young Diane decided then and there that she someday wanted a large family. By the time she married Tom, the love of her life, she decided maybe 6 children was a better number than 12. She enjoys her life in southwestern Ohio with Tom and their six children. Two daughters, Christina and April, live away from home with successful careers. Two other children, Bartholomew and Emily, are attending college. Life is never boring with two daughters, Sara and Amanda, born with Down Syndrome, living at home. Tom is very supportive of Diane's writing career as well as their awesome children.*

Diane writes inspirational romance, mainstream, chick-lit mystery, nonfiction, and articles. No Greater Loss *and* A Fiery Secret *are available in print at Borders and Waldenbooks.* Never the Same *is available as an ebook and will be released in print in August 2007. All three books are published by Samhain and can also be purchased at mybookstoreandmore.com. Diane's other books,* The Christmas of 1957, *and* Celebrating and Caring for Your Baby With Special Needs *are available at booklocker.com.* How to Run A Profitable Preschool *is in ebook format and is also available at booklocker.com.*

11. Delivery by Pony Express
by Jodi W.

Vaginal, caesarean...my first child could have been delivered by pony express for all I cared. For eight months, my precious baby had been treated to a caffeine-free, alcohol-free, secondhand smoke-free mommy. However, there was one thing I couldn't protect my baby from—Tegretol, the anticonvulsant medication I took four times a day for a seizure disorder I'd had since childhood. Although there hadn't been any studies for my specific medication, the doctors seemed optimistic even though they admitted an increased chance of birth defects.

I chose not to think about the possibilities. If I *never* thought about or discussed the negative outcomes, they just wouldn't happen, right? That worked for eight months, until my water broke exactly one month before my due date. All the possibilities loomed before me and I was certain something was wrong with my beautiful baby. So, when my husband and I arrived at the hospital and learned that, not only was the baby in breech position, but I was also at 10 cm after two measly contractions, I didn't care about the c-section. All those people scurrying around the operating room only enforced my negativity. "Something's wrong they aren't telling me," I thought just before the anesthesiologist placed the mask over my face and asked me to count backwards.

When my husband told me about our perfect little daughter in the recovery room, I thought my worries were over. Unfortunately, I was just trading them in for a new set of problems. As my husband marveled about our tiny handful of a baby, not even six pounds, I replied by throwing up all over his shoes. Nausea caused by the general anesthesia would be a minor inconvenience for most women. For me, it was a full-blown disaster. Not only was I unable to keep down crackers, cereal, or even juice, but also the anti-convulsant medication I relied on. The first seizure happened was when I was introducing my newborn to my teenage brother. He held his niece for the first time when he grabbed her away from me.

I only remember brief glimpses after that. The hospital's neurologist finally stopped the seizures by giving me a high dose of Dilantin, an anti-convulsant that left me 'doped up'. My frantic family finally managed to get my neurologist and the hospital's neurologist communicating and, after a long week in the hospital, my nausea, seizures, and 'high' were all gone.

I swore I would never return to that hospital or obstetrician. When I was pregnant 3 years later, I decided to travel to a hospital and high-risk obstetrician 45 minutes from our house, even though there was another local hospital and other local obstetricians. When my doctor asked about my birthing plan, it was simple: no c-section, no drugs, nothing that might cause a repeat of that nightmare week. I'd like to say I chose that birthing plan because I wanted to experience a natural birth, bond with my newborn, and do what was best for my baby. But truthfully, I was afraid. Some women choose a planned caesarean section because they're afraid of the pain. I chose *not* to have a caesarean section because I was afraid of seizures. There was no reluctance to my VBAC plan from the doctors or hospital; it was treated as standard operating procedure.

This time, my labor began even earlier, six weeks before my due date, but with a short hospital stay and three weeks of bed rest we managed to hold my eager daughter off for three more weeks. When we were settling into the labor/delivery room and the nurse asked about my pain management plan, I emphatically insisted that I was not taking any medication. She dutifully wrote it on my chart but there was a "Yeah, we'll see" glint in her eye. But with a determination spurred on by fear, I labored without any medical relief except a topical pain reliever just before delivery. Thankfully, our daughter arrived only two hours after we walked into the maternity ward. My memories of my first glimpse of her are not clouded by drugs, or post-seizure haziness. There was no nausea to make me too weak to hold her. I was able to leave the hospital and return to my cozy home and my family less than 48 hours after delivery. I was sold on VBAC!

I would have been happy to return to my VBAC hospital and obstetrician for my third pregnancy but there were other things to consider. My pregnancies and deliveries had become increasingly shorter—could I manage a 45-minute ride to the hospital or would I be delivering my baby on some lonely stretch of country road? My baby was due in mid-March, which meant I would be traveling to doctor's appointments (that would become a weekly chore because of my history of pre-term labor) throughout an entire Pennsylvania winter. What happened if there was a blizzard? Would I end up at our local hospital delivering with the help of a doctor I had never met before, someone who might not want to attempt a VBAC delivery?

I called my cousin, a nursery nurse at the local hospital (*not* the one where I delivered my oldest daughter). Tearfully, I asked her if any of the local obstetricians were any good. Could they deal with my problems? Would they force me to have a c-section? Once again, pregnancy had made me afraid—not of pain, but of seizures. But MJ promised me that things had changed in our small community in the eleven years since my first daughter was born. She knew just the doctor for me. I would come to her hospital; she and her fellow nurses would take care of me.

> *I don't think an initial choice or necessity should compel a woman to a lifetime of caesarean sections.*

Between my history of pre-term labor and my seizure condition, my obstetrician had enough on her mind. VBAC wasn't even an issue. Once again, it was standard operating procedure. I started out planning a repeat of my younger daughter's birth but my cousin and doctor introduced me to the possibility of an epidural, something that wasn't even available with my first child. But I was still frightened of any medical procedures when I arrived at the labor/delivery room after a nerve-wracking two months of early labor, bed rest, and three visits to the hospital (one during a snowstorm).

My cousin, with the determination our family is famous (infamous?) for, finally convinced me that an epidural and general anesthesia were world's apart. I consented to "curl your back like a stretching cat"—something I couldn't even manage to do when I didn't have a pulsating basketball for a stomach. Somehow, my cat imitation worked, the epidural was administered, and I promptly announced that I wanted to kiss the anesthesiologist. It had taken me 11 years to get over the fear I associated with birthing medical procedures. Not long after that, I welcomed my son into the world with a surprised, "He's so big!" He continues to surprise me every day.

I would never change the circumstances of my older daughter's birth because I believe the c-section was necessary for a safe delivery. But, I don't think an initial choice or necessity should compel a woman to a lifetime of caesarean sections. To some degree, past birth experiences should be considered. Perhaps if one VBAC attempt had resulted in tearing of a c-section scar, it should be ruled out for subsequent births. But, barring serious problems such as that, I believe each birth should be considered independently. I would hate to have the memory of an anesthesia mask coming down over my face to be my only memory of the birth experience.

Jodi W. is the mother of two daughters, ages 14 and 11, and one 3-year-old son. She is thankful that, among her large, extended family, she has one strong-willed nurse who showed up on her day off to help deliver a beautiful boy. Jodi also writes for a variety of magazines, including Toy Directory Monthly, Birds and Blooms, *and* The History Magazine.

12. Two Successful VBACs
by Brenda Ruggiero

My first child – a son – was delivered by cesarean in 1993. Like many first-time parents, my husband and I had gone through childbirth classes. They went over what would happen if we had to have a cesarean, but we never expected that we would be in that category.

My water broke almost a month before my due date and, when we went to the hospital, my doctor decided to induce labor, since I hadn't started having any contractions yet. After several hours of monitoring, he determined that there was fetal distress, since the baby's heart rate went down even during small contractions. He decided to deliver by cesarean. The cord was around my son's neck, and there was a knot in it. But, he was perfectly healthy and never had any problems. I am still thankful that the doctor made the decision that he did.

Baby number two was due when my first son was just over 2-1/2 years old in 1996. I went to the same doctor, who happened to have a new partner at this time. I felt very comfortable with both of them. We discussed my options for delivery, and they encouraged me to try a vaginal delivery. Then they left the final decision up to my husband and me. We could opt for a repeat cesarean or attempt a vaginal birth.

I did as much research as I could to determine what my decision should be. At that time, I did not have Internet access (something I can't imagine now!), so it was more difficult to conduct research. But, my sister worked for the county health department, and she was able to get me some articles to read. Most of what I read was pro-VBAC, but my husband and I decided that we would opt for a C-section because of the risks involved.

My change of heart came about during my seventh month. It seems rather silly now to think about it, but it happened when I was watching, of all things, a soap opera. During a scene where a woman delivers a baby

We knew that this baby was a gift from God, and we trusted that He would bring it safely into the world, regardless of the method. Our God doesn't rely on statistics to do His work!

in an elevator, something clicked within me. I realized that if I didn't at least attempt to have a vaginal delivery this time, I would probably never know what it was like to give birth the way women have done it since the beginning of time. After some explaining, my husband supported me in my decision, and we told the doctor what I wanted to do.

My faith was also an important part of this decision. We knew that this baby was a gift from God, and we trusted that He would bring it safely into the world, regardless of the method. Our God doesn't rely on statistics to do His work! So we prayed and trusted.

I was advised to come to the hospital early in my labor so I could be monitored, and was also encouraged to have an epidural, which would make it easy for them to quickly do a cesarean if needed. Like most women I know, I didn't have to be told twice to get the epidural!

Everything went smoothly with both labor and delivery. The doctor did have to use suction to get the baby out (another debate in itself) but, other than that, there were no complications for me, or for the baby. Our second son arrived by successful VBAC, with the added bonus of being a leap year baby!

When I got pregnant for the third time, I was disappointed to discover that my doctor had retired and I had to find a new one. However, I was pleased with the one I found. There was no question that I would attempt a second vaginal birth, and he supported that decision.

Once more, I had no complications, and my daughter was born vaginally in 1999. This labor went much faster, and there was no time for an epidural. But I survived the ordeal, as many women do, and had no problems.

Brenda Ruggiero is a freelance writer from western Maryland.

13. Induced At Home—
A Midwife Uses Cytotec
by Karen Putz

Meet my son, Steven, a lanky 8-year-old who loves to play basketball with his older brother. With a mess of dirty blonde hair, strangers often come up and comment on his beautiful eyes and gentle grin. The youngest of my trio of kids, Steven was born at home, a VBAC after two cesareans.

While a home birth after two cesareans is becoming a rarity nowadays, what's unusual about his birth is that he was induced.

The midwife used Cytotec.

Cytotec, otherwise known as Misoprostol, is a medicine that is used to prevent or treat ulcers. It is FDA approved for this use only, but caregivers have discovered that in doses of 25 and 50 micrograms, Cytotec can bring on labor. The pill is often obtained in doses of 100 micrograms and cut in half or quarters to obtain a smaller dosage. The pill is either taken orally or inserted vaginally to start labor.

Shortly after my second child was born by c-section, I experienced a lot of sadness about her birth. I knew that I didn't want to have another hospital birth and I began to explore the home birth option. I read several books about home birth and books about VBAC. I contacted one of the VBAC

> *Shortly after my second child was born by c-section, I experienced a lot of sadness about her birth.*

> *I certainly didn't expect a chemical induction to be a part of midwifery.*

authors, who gave me a referral to "one of the best midwives." The midwife was quoted as having a 100 percent VBAC record.

Impressed, my husband and I made contact and drove up to meet her. As someone who was very new to midwifery, I dove headfirst into it. In some ways, I still hadn't learned to trust myself, choosing instead to place my trust in the midwifery model of care. I certainly didn't expect a chemical induction to be a part of midwifery. Even at the first visit, however, the idea of using Cytotec came up. The name wasn't used; I was simply told that she and her midwife partners had a pill that successfully started labor. Because I lived six hours away, the midwives were originally going to have me take the pill home and insert it into my cervix so that I would be in labor when they arrived.

The more I thought about it, the more I realized my apprehensions about the pill. I called the midwife and expressed my concerns about safety. She reassured me and said—and I quote—"It's perfectly safe." I figured that she and her partners had far more experience than I did, and I trusted them, just as I had earlier with my doctors. To make a long story short, the midwives arrived around my due date and Cytotec was inserted. I was told it would take about three hours for labor to begin.

About five hours later, labor kicked in. I experienced back labor during transition and it was really intense. Because I supposedly had a low pubic arch and the baby in a compound position, I ended up "alley-ooped" in the McRobert's position with my knees up to my ears, fundal pressure applied twice after a mere 10 minutes of pushing, and my baby torqued out. I was told I had a normal birth.

For the longest time after Steven's birth, I had nothing but praise for the midwives who attended. After all, there were many wonderful memories of being served dinner and breakfast, laundry being done and words of encouragement being spoken. There was the ultimate triumph of birthing vaginally after two cesareans. And surely midwives would never use an intervention unless it was necessary, I reminded myself. After all, they're the experts in normal, natural childbirth. Aren't they?

When my baby was a couple months old, we purchased a computer. Little by little, I started learning more about Cytotec. I learned about all the niggling side effects that my midwives neglected to mention, such as ruptures, hyper-stimulation of the uterus, fetal distress and fetal death. One site that listed the side effects had a warning: *This drug is not to be used on pregnant women!* I learned that Cytotec was definitely not recommended for women with prior uterine surgery.

Thank goodness I had the uterus of steel, as a fellow International Cesarean Awareness Network (ICAN) member once said.

I wrote to my midwives, sending studies and asking questions about the interventions. I was basically told that, without them, I would have ended up with another cesarean. As for the Cytotec, I was told, "The only side effect of Cytotec is maternal contractions." I was also told to quit second-guessing and to "lighten up."

Lighten up?

I became angry instead.

I was angry that I naively exposed my son to something that is highly experimental and with risk. I was also sad and dismayed to find other midwives using Cytotec in home births. All the books that I read in preparation for home birth described midwife as attendants who let nature take its course and as experts in natural birth. That is the ultimate betrayal—to plan a home birth, hire a midwife and end up with obstetrics at home. Without Internet access, nothing prepared me for the medicalization of Steven's birth.

For a long time, I held on to that anger. I found other women who had birthed with the same midwife and had medicalized births as well. Meeting the other moms in person and via the Internet set a healing process in motion.

I met another mom on the Internet who lived near me and was planning a home birth after two cesareans. She invited me to her home birth and I was able to support her when her daughter was born in a pool of warm water. That special home birth was a healing that allowed me to finally let go of the anger that I was carrying around.

Karen Putz is a mom to three deaf and hard of hearing children. She is a board member of Hands & Voices National (http://www.handsandvoices.org) and works in early intervention. Karen also teaches Conversational Sign Language at a local community college.

14. VBA2C: VBAC After Two Cesareans!
by Deana Atherton

It was the steamy New York summer of 2005 as I awaited the arrival of my much-anticipated fifth child. My husband and I were beyond thrilled to be pregnant again and welcome a new baby into our family. My only worries centered around whether or not I would succeed in my quest for a vaginal birth after two cesareans (VBA2C). The road to success was a LONG and winding one, filled with many bumps and uncertainties. But, in the end, I was triumphant. On July 28, 2005 at 9:04 pm, I gave birth to a gorgeous, healthy baby girl and I succeeded in having my much anticipated VBA2C!!

Madeleine's was my fifth pregnancy. My first two were normal and uneventful, yet beautiful vaginal deliveries. My third baby was a c-section due to transverse presentation. Reluctantly, on my end, I agreed to a repeat c-section with my fourth baby at my OB's insistence. I was determined to do my research and have a strong voice in my next baby's birth!! Immediately upon testing positive on a home pregnancy test, I knew with every fiber of my being that I was going on a quest for a VBA2C. Little did I know then that calling it a quest was putting it mildy!

I had to search with all my energies to find a provider on Long Island, NY willing to do a VBA2C. I was turned away by several candidates before I found my midwife. She was a tremendous blessing every step of the way. With all of her heart and soul, she knew I could do this. She never doubted me for a minute and she supported and encouraged me when I doubted myself. She believed in my body's ability to give birth and in my right to have a voice in determining how my baby entered this world.

She told me to listen to my body, listen to my inner voice, trust my instincts and believe all would turn out fine. She was right.

On the night of July 27th, I was one day past due and I decided to have my membranes stripped by one of the midwives in the office. A few hours later, in the middle of the night, I had some pretty decent contractions. I was excited as I tossed and turned in bed, thinking perhaps this was the night. Unfortunately, when I got up to shower the following morning, the contractions had stopped. But things were happening! I took my two little boys to the park early that afternoon and as they played happily in the sand, I contemplated drinking an Alice-in-Wonderland-type concoction for labor induction. A good friend had told me about a castor oil milk shake recipe with eggs[14] - a midwives' secret formula for inducing labor without the discomfort and embarrassment of the accompanying diarrhea. After hashing out the pros and cons on the park bench, the blazing sun got the better of me. The little "drink me" sign was calling my name! I took my little boys home, almost hastily made the castor oil milkshake in my blender, and drank it before I could change my mind!

I felt totally fine and normal for the first couple of hours after drinking the shake. Then, around 4:15, I felt like I should lie down. I just felt a little off, a little queasy perhaps. I thought the castor oil was just making me nauseated. My mother was visiting and, at about 4:30 or so, said she was going to leave. I got up to walk her to the door at 4:45 and, boom, had my first real contraction. I figured I had plenty of time so my mother left anyway. Luckily, my husband was there working from home, hoping I would go into labor. From that moment on, the contractions did not let up. They were strong, frequent, and

---

[14] *Pregnant women are advised not to take home remedies without the approval and guidance of their healthcare provider. As mentioned in a previous chapter, castor oil can be very dangerous.*

very consistent right from the beginning! (No diarrhea though!!) My husband timed them for me and it was readily apparent we needed to call my sister to come over and watch

> *I want mothers to know it can be done. And it can be done safely and beautifully.*

the children until we could get my parents back over. I began to worry and stress about the potential for uterine rupture with each pain. I sat on the toilet in the bathroom as my husband dialed the on-call midwife. When I got on the phone, I expressed my angst about rupturing. I knew the odds were in my favor. I had done my research to the point of delirium, but I was not feeling very rational at that moment. She very clearly said to me, "I'm not worried about your uterus rupturing. I'm worried you're not going to get to the hospital in time."

That was all my husband needed to hear. Knowing the traffic in New York as well as we do, and having to drive during rush-hour, we knew we better get in high gear ASAP.

The ride was agony. The contractions were very intense, pretty regular, anywhere from four to five minutes apart, to two minutes apart. The traffic was bumper-to-bumper for the majority of the 40-minute ride. My saving grace was the cool washcloth my sweet daughter gave me before I got in the car to leave. That silly little washcloth helped me more than anything during the whole labor experience! I think the fact that she gave it to me gave it its special soothing properties. When we finally pulled up to the hospital, I was mortified. My husband left me halfway out of the car door to go get a wheel chair inside while hundreds of people were walking by the traffic circle. There was more embarrassment as I went in to be checked and there was no available room. I had to labor in the waiting room, probably frightening half to death the poor couple that was sitting there watching television! By the time a room was available and they checked me, I was 4cm and 80% effaced.

(Ugh! Only four??) I remember mouthing "help me" to my husband every time the midwife looked away. I can't help it. What can I say? I get desperate in labor! Things progressed quickly after that. By the time I got into the labor and delivery room, it was about 7:30 or 7:45. I was begging for an epidural pretty immediately. My birth ball and a hot shower did not at all seem like viable or comfortable options to me. I wanted immediate gratification! I did get the epidural but, unfortunately, it did not take effect. I think I may have been too far dilated at that point because, truthfully, it did not lessen the pain more than taking the faintest edge off of it. The on-call midwife was nothing short of amazing. She told my husband to go find my sister and have her come into the labor room! What a surprise! I was so happy and so relieved to see her. Having my sister and my sweet husband there truly did help me work through the pain (that and my washcloth which my husband and the nurse kept wetting for me repeatedly).

Suddenly, I felt a pop and a gush of warmth and wetness at about 8:50 or so. My midwife ran over with a sense of urgency and checked my progress. I was fully dilated and fully effaced! She gently guided me as I panted and pushed my sweet baby out into the world. After six minutes and only a handful or so of pushes, Madeleine Eve was born. All warm and wet and slippery, this beautiful child slid out and was placed on my chest. I'll never forget the feeling of her body on mine, or her big blue eyes as she glanced up at me for the first time.

And, I'll never forget the look of pure joy and peace on my husband's face as he watched our newest daughter enter the world. It is a moment I will treasure and carry with me always, a moment I thought I would never again experience after having two c-sections. I want mothers to know it can be done. And it can be done safely and beautifully. This birth was so incredibly healing for me, allowing me to release the anger and frustration I have felt over my c-section experiences.

After Madeleine's birth, the midwife dimmed the lights so I could hold my baby in a peaceful, soothing environment. I held her, as did my husband and my sister, for what felt like hours. I nursed her and she latched on immediately. We were not rushed. The whole experience was nothing short of magical. When the baby did finally have to go up to the nursery, we sat in pow-wow like fashion talking, laughing, reliving the birth ~ my midwife, my sister, my husband, the nurse, and me sitting cross-legged on the bed I had just given birth in. I could not help but feel so blessed to be experiencing a celebration of life reminiscent of births from a bygone era, unhurried, relaxed, blissfully happy, just soaking in the natural high that this birth had brought to all who experienced it.

Unforgettable....

Deana is a stay at home mom to five wonderful children. She has her teaching certification and masters in Teaching English to Speakers of Other Languages, which she looks forward to using when the children are all in school full-time. She enjoys hiking, yoga, writing, going to the beach, and vacationing with her family.

15. I Fired My OB at 35 Weeks
by L.S.

When I was a first time mom, I did no reading up on pregnancy except for maybe *What to Expect While You're Expecting* and occasional viewings of *A Baby Story* on television. My mom had 3 kids vaginally and my grandma had 15.

I went to a six-doctor group practice. I had a checkup at 39 weeks, 3 days. It was the first one my husband had gotten to attend with me. He works third shift and the appointment was at 8:30. Of course, I didn't even get into the exam room until 9:30. Everyone was making a big deal about the fact that my blood pressure was a tad high, around 146/82 at the office. I think I had my blood pressure checked four times before going to the hospital. (When I checked my hospital records before my VBAC, I found it ironic that my blood pressure was perfectly fine except for when it and my child's heart rate plummeted after the administration of the epidural. Ephedrine was administered and saved me from an emergency c-section at that time.)

Immediately after my vaginal exam, I stood up to get dressed and my water started gushing. The doc said he wanted me to go to the hospital because of my blood pressure. In retrospect, I think he stripped my membranes and accidentally broke my water during my exam.

> In retrospect, I think he stripped my membranes and accidentally broke my water during my exam.

When I got there, I was denied food because I "might throw up". My records later indicated that I'd been at one point allowed clear liquids or ice chips, but no one pushed them on me. During the labor, I had Nubian, an epidural, Pitocin, and finally felt the urge to push around 3 a.m., about 17 hours after my membranes ruptured. I pushed the best I could. I couldn't feel contractions very well because of the epidural and was tired because I'd been awake almost

> *I started crying and said, "I don't want a c-section!"*
>
> *The doctor laughed and said, "L, no one WANTS a c-section."*

24 hours. I was desperately thirsty and had been without anything to drink for almost 24 hours, too.

The doctor came in at one time and yelled at my husband when he sat down in between contractions. They had me in what midwives know as the worst position for pushing: flat on the back, or stranded beetle, with a nurse holding one leg and my husband holding the other. My husband had been awake for almost 40 hours and yelling at him in front of me didn't help. Both my and the nurse's jaws dropped and she was the first to defend him and then me. I was really starting to feel tired and starting to say, "I can't."

I remember the nurses saying they could see my child's brown hair. The doctor did an episiotomy and vacuum and then told me that I'd pushed for a little over two hours and, if I didn't have her out by then, it probably wasn't going to happen.

I said, "Can't we try something else?"

She asked me, "What would you have me try?"

I asked about changing my position and was told, "No."

I started crying and said, "I don't want a c-section!"

The doctor laughed and said, "L, no one WANTS a c-section."

Seven days after admitted, I went home. Both the baby and I developed a fever in the hospital. So, antibiotics for us and a nice case of thrush for her when she got home. I went home feeling like I was run over by a truck. I was taking 1025 milligrams of iron for almost transfusion level blood loss. Despite that colon-clogging amount of iron, I developed symptoms that I recognized from working in a nursing home as "c-diff". Imagine having loose, green, uncontrollable stools for about a month... I had to put my screaming daughter down in her bed twice to clean myself up and finally resorted to Depends® for a while.

Whenever I called the doctor's office, I was told it was just the hormones and drugs working their way out of my system. "Take Jello® water and Immodium®".

At the checkup, the doctor told me that she'd put in my OR report that my pelvis was suitable for a 9lb child. She told me that my c-section was just "one of those things". She again promised I could try VBAC the next time, like she promised at the hospital before my c-section.

Despite that horrible birth experience, I stayed with that OB group, seeing their nurses for pap smears. About 3½ years later, we decided to try to conceive and did so immediately. While on a trip to the library with my child, I noticed the book *The VBAC Companion* by Diana Korte, and checked it out. After reading it, I had an appointment at 33 weeks with the same doc who'd sent me to the hospital over three years earlier with ruptured membranes. While measuring my belly, he asked me how large my first child had been. 7lb., 12 oz.

He said, "You grow them big". He then whistled when he heard my husband had been a 10 lb baby.

I asked him a question I'd seen in Diana Korte's book, "What are my chances of VBAC?"

> When I asked him about a doula, he said, "Not necessary".

He made a motion of looking over my OR report and said, "Well, your first child was so big. Unless you get lucky and have her early, you'll probably have to have a section with this one too."

I could hardly look at him because I knew what his partner had told me about 9 lbs and I wasn't really impressed with someone that would say "lucky" and "early baby" in the same sentence. When I asked him about a doula, he said, "Not necessary".

I contacted a local birth resource center for advice and names of possible doulas. The director suggested I get my hospital records. When I did I was just SHOCKED. It was full of charting about how my husband was unsympathetic and said the c-section had been done at +3 pelvic station with fetal and maternal vitals reassuring. I knew that our vitals were fine at the time, but when the doctor said she didn't think I could push out my child, I assumed she knew she was talking about.

She'd been to more births than me. The books I was reading had pelvic chart pictures and I knew +3 was right there. After I had my VBAC, I found this quote[15] on the Internet from a book by Gerard M. DiLeo, M.D., F.A.C.O.G:

> "+3 is 3 cm below the ischial spines, and, well, you better call the doctor, because that baby's about to deliver! True, a +3 station shows the baby's scalp on the perineum (at the opening of the vagina)"

My doc had decided +3 meant to do a c-section.

---

[15] See: http://www.gynob.com/ggstation.htm

I hired a doula who had no VBAC experience, but with whom I clicked. She suggested home birth. I met with the woman who delivered her first and only child. She was a VBA2C mom herself and handled VBAC clients. In the end, we both turned each other down. I was scared of the "what ifs" and she said I didn't seem to believe in home birth enough. I'd also interviewed her back-up OB and he commented on how most moms who home birthed were sure about their decision, but I was not sure. The midwife believed that this OB believed in vaginal birth and having a supportive caregiver was half the battle. So, at 35 weeks, I asked for my records to be switched to a new doctor. I got a call from a secretary at my old OB's office, but refused to tell her why I switched. Part of me was afraid that Dr. S. was right about my first child being too big, and I really didn't need the mental anguish of debating with them. I just insisted it was my decision and that was that.

I had a checkup at 40 weeks, 2 days (Friday) and I think both the doc and I were disappointed to find I was only dilated to "maybe two centimeters."

On Monday, I awoke at 5 a.m. with contractions. I called the doula around noon. I tried resting, but couldn't, so I took a long shower to help with pain. (I think I ended up with two or three showers before my baby was born.)

We tried timing contractions, but couldn't with the distraction of my oldest child. My husband took her over to her grandmother's at 7 p.m., about the same time I was expecting the doula. She had me walk around the neighborhood several times. She reminded me to eat and drink. She had me going up and down the stairs two at a time and doing lunges. She had me in the shower again. She was concerned that my contractions weren't long enough to dilate my cervix. They were short, but close together. She even suggested I needed to call my doctor to see if he had any ideas on getting my labor going. I refused because I didn't want to be put on the clock[16].

> *In retrospect, I think it's true what I've heard that, if left alone, a VBAC mom's body will labor in a way to protect her.*

Sometime during the night, I had some classic signs of "transition": feeling cold and then hot and vomiting, but the short contractions had everyone snowed. When my water broke around 3 a.m. on Tuesday, I agreed to let the doula call my doc and he asked that we go to the hospital. While going through the admittance stuff and the placing of the IV, I had the feeling I wanted to push and started moaning, "No push."

Finally, I asked them to check me and two nurses did it. I have the feeling the first nurse couldn't believe what she found. I was 10 cm and totally effaced with the rest of my water sack bulging. When the doc got there and they told him, he looked kind of shocked and said, "Well, now our job is to help her deliver this baby."

Some things were just the same as my first labor. I was in labor and awake for almost 24 hours. I pushed for two hours again. Some things were so different. I was allowed drink while pushing. I felt I had more support. In the end, I pushed out our 8 lb, 9 oz daughter 6 days after my due date.

In retrospect, I think it's true what I've heard that, if left alone, a VBAC mom's body will labor in a way to protect her. Thus, my short contractions. Also, I have decided that, since I was so

---

[16] *Some physicians and hospitals give laboring women time limits to meet certain milestones, such as a certain number of hours to dilate to 10 cm and to push. If the woman doesn't meet these milestones, she may be subjected to unnecessary medical intervention.*

afraid to go to the hospital, I'll just skip going to the hospital and stay home with a midwife if I ever have another baby.

L.S. is a stay at home mom from Indiana to two daughters, ages six and two. She's been married to her college sweetheart for 10 years.

16. A Birth I Can Dream About Now
by Robyn Morton

My VBAC story starts with a c-section for "failure to progress". In the recovery room, I was told by the attending nurse that I should never attempt a vaginal birth because the risks were just too great. Not even an hour after my birth, I was heartbroken. I had no idea until that moment that I'd lost my chance to have a normal birth. However, my doctor said that there was no reason I couldn't attempt a vaginal birth in the future. I was confused by this contradictory information, as well as depressed about my birth. I began researching VBACs. I also began attending a c-section support group. Ironically, I had one of the smoothest physical recoveries one could hope for, but the mental recovery has taken years.

Two years later, we conceived again. The decision to try for a VBAC was both very easy and very difficult for me. On the one hand, I knew I wanted to try to have a vaginal birth; I wanted the experience of "giving birth" rather than of "having birth done to me". But the risks of a VBAC weighed heavily on my mind, complicated by my worries that I was so desperate for a vaginal birth that I was jeopardizing the safety of myself and our baby. We researched the risks of both VBACs and repeat c-sections extensively. By the end of my research, I had decided that not only is VBAC the safer route, but that the hospital environment—with its laundry list of interventions—might pose a greater risk to me than the VBAC itself.

Ironically, I had one of the smoothest physical recoveries one could hope for, but the mental recovery has taken years.

143

When I was six months pregnant, we moved to Alabama and found a supportive doctor. I was still uncomfortable with the idea of a hospital birth, though. I began researching home birth. I became increasingly convinced that being at home would not only greatly improve my chances of a successful vaginal birth, but would also be the safer environment in which to give birth. We found a midwife and a doula, and began planning a home birth, while maintaining my OB appointments so that transporting to the hospital would go smoothly if something went wrong.

The pregnancy itself was almost entirely uneventful. I was due on December 6th, and so the Christmas newborn outfits started rolling in. My due date passed without a flutter, but we remained unconcerned, if anxious. I knew that the 40-week due date is only a rough estimate, and that we had another 2 weeks to go before anyone should be concerned. At 41 weeks, my doctor informed me that he would be going on Christmas vacation the following week. While he was optimistic that I would begin labor before this, he wanted to discuss scheduling non-stress tests and ultrasounds for 41.5 weeks as a sort of "pre-emptive" measure, in case any of the other doctors would try and push me into an unwanted induction while he was away. The tests all came out fine, so we were content to wait.

Unfortunately, so was the baby. What proceeded from this point can only be described as a comedy of errors. On Dec. 19th, everyone thought I had begun labor. The midwife brought in her equipment. We put a lasagna in the oven for everyone, and settled in for a long night. My labor never intensified, though, and by the next morning it was clear that it was petering out. The next day, we had an exceedingly unpleasant visit with a new OB. He used scare tactic statements such as "big baby" to frighten us into a c-section. My husband responded with concerns about iatrogenic complications[17] caused by inductions. It is remarkable how quickly a doctor will change his demeanor when a patient starts using terms like "iatrogenic" (i.e., doctor-caused). We scheduled more tests in three days and left to meet with our midwife. She was becoming uncomfortable with us attempting a home birth (as were we). We agreed that Wednesday would be our cut-off date. If my labor had not begun by then, she would come over in the morning and break my water to see if we could jumpstart labor. If so, we would proceed with a home birth; if not, we would head for the hospital to discuss our options with the doctor on call.

Between the days of Sunday and Wednesday, our only car broke down, I developed a raging head cold, our doula went out of town for Christmas and our midwife developed severe pneumonia. There were no other midwives in the area that we trusted, and so our home birth plan was at an end. Obviously, someone was trying to get us to go to the hospital, so off we went.

When we arrived at the hospital, we were feeling depressed and defeated. We were worried that we were heading down exactly the same road that resulted in a c-section last time. However, at the nurses station was a nurse from our church who had wanted to apprentice under our midwife and attend our home birth. She knew that we'd wanted a home birth, and did everything she could to help us have the birth we'd been hoping for. Just seeing a friendly, familiar face at the hospital

---

[17] *"An iatrogenic complication is an unfavorable response to medical treatment that is induced by the therapeutic effort itself. Although some are minor, others are life-threatening. Serious or fatal iatrogenic complications occur in 4 to 9 percent of hospitalized patients."*
Source: http://www.usalaw.com/a-mm-iatrogenic-complications-medical-care.html

went a long way towards me being more comfortable in an otherwise scary environment.

We talked with the doctor and agreed to try breaking my water and walking for a few hours to see if that would start labor. I did start contracting, but not in a good pattern, so we decided to go ahead and try a low dose of Pitocin[18], rather than going for a repeat c-section right away. During my walking, I did progress from 4 to 5 cm., so I was optimistic that my body was ready. After a few hours of Pitocin and good contractions, though, I was still at 5 cm. Brian and I were becoming depressed, sure that I would stall and end up in surgery again. However, the doctor was very calm and reassuring. He pointed out that the baby was doing fine, and that delivering in an hour via c-section or at 2 a.m. vaginally made no difference to him, so I wasn't under much time pressure. I decided that if I had not made any progress in another couple of hours, I would request an epidural; I hoped that having pain relief would allow me to relax and finish dilating. When I was checked an hour later, I'd made it to 7 cm., and decided to decline the epidural—my mobility was too important to give up easily. I kept going but I was beginning to fight the contractions—balling up and tensing, dreading every new one. I was checked in two more hours and was still at seven cm. so I asked for the epidural. Apparently, though, the anesthesiologist had gone home, so they had to call him back, which would take time.

The anesthesiologist was not happy about having to leave his home again, and over the Christmas holidays. I suppose that's

---

[18] *WARNING - Pitocin and other labor-inducing/enhancing drugs increase the chance of uterine rupture. Many doctors now refuse to give these drugs to women who are attempting a VBAC. Do not allow your doctor to administer these drugs until reading about the possible life threatening results. See: http://www.home birth.org.uk/pe2.htm*

why he did a bad job. When I first got the epidural I thought I'd entered heaven. I could still feel the contractions, but barely, and the pain had finally ended, at least for the next hour or so. My epidural mysteriously stopped working—pretty soon the only thing that was numb were my legs. No one was sure what to do, and the anesthesiologist was gone again. I was incoherent. Pitocin-induced transitional labor is a terrible experience. If they couldn't fix my epidural, I'd decided I would rip the IV out of my arm to make it stop. The anesthesiologist finally called back to give a new dosage for the epidural. The epidural never gave me good pain relief again, but it at least made the breaks between contractions real, which was what I needed.

Since I had an epidural in place, my desires to push in various positions went out the window—it's hard to squat when you have no control over your legs. This was frustrating, as I could tell that my body really *wanted* to be upright, I just couldn't do it. So, there I was in the stirrups like I'd sworn I'd never do. Even with the epidural, though, I was able to push fairly effectively. I never did have an urge to push, because that was being blocked by the epidural, but I could feel the contractions and pushed through them.

At one point, the doctor asked how long I thought I'd been pushing and I responded, "I don't know, about 20 minutes maybe?" I looked at the clock and found that it had been over two hours, and the baby still kept sliding back up after every push. I was getting worn out, and the OB suggested that we use a vacuum extractor to at least get the baby past this sticking point. I agreed, and we spent another 30 minutes pushing and pulling. Finally, the baby was crowning, but I was pretty exhausted. The OB said, "I know you don't want an episiotomy, but I really think it'll help." I agreed, and he made the cut. Of all the things that happened, this is the only decision

I really regret; I wish I'd asked for another two or three pushes—I'm confident he would have agreed.

Finally, the head was out, then one shoulder, then the next, but I still had to push hard. He didn't "slip out" until it was only his legs left! This was perhaps because he weighed 9 lbs., 14 oz.—definitely not a small baby. I had to smirk, though, since my c-section report said that my pelvis was too small. This baby was over two pounds heavier than my last, and bigger in every way. If I had not been restricted to pushing on my back, I'm confident that he would have come out much more smoothly. They put the baby on my chest and he didn't leave there for the next two hours, except to be weighed. That time with my husband, mom, and new baby was worth it all.

At the end of the day, I'd submitted to practically every medical practice that I didn't want but, once it was all over, I was a happy camper. I was happy because my husband and I had felt in control of the process. We understood the interventions being used, and we agreed with them. We knew when we needed to say no. We had strategies for how to employ the interventions available. We never felt bullied. I don't know how I would have felt if I'd ended up with another c-section, but I do know that I would not have suffered the two years of mental trauma I did after my first one. My VBAC wasn't the birth of my dreams, but it was a birth I can dream about now.

Robyn Morton was born and raised in a small town on the outskirts of St. Louis, Missouri. She has a Bachelor's degree in French and Philosophy & Religion, and a Master's in Philosophy. She lived in Seattle for a time, pursuing her PhD in Philosophy, but life intervened. She is married to her college boyfriend, who is also a philosopher. She has been a waitress, childcare provider, housekeeper, office assistant, teaching assistant, computer tech support person, and line chef. She is now a stay-at-home mom, an amateur gardener, an overenthusiastic home cook, an armchair policy theorist, a birth activist, a backseat philosopher for her husband, and a semi-rabid proponent of sustainable living with a penchant for permaculture.

17. Position and the Right Support Mean Everything
by Wendy Bat-Sarah

For my first labor, I was induced over a completely unripe cervix. I experienced contractions for about eight hours, then lost heart and got an epidural, which almost immediately caused fetal distress. The distress never really cleared up and, about two hours after the epidural, I had a c-section.

It is Friday, March 12th, the day after my 33rd birthday. I'm starting to feel pressured. The midwives have scheduled me for an appointment with the back-up doctor (my due date was the 7th), and one of them keeps talking about how huge this baby is going to be. Another one keeps talking about how horribly high my blood pressure is (in fact, it isn't).

I start contemplating doing castor oil and other drastic things. I just want this over with. Two of my friends remind me that I've spent all this time and effort learning to trust my body's wisdom—that it would be silly to lose faith so late in the game. I wrote out a bunch of affirmations—all about how I could move into and through the pain—how everyone else was here simply to help *me* get what *I* needed.

Shortly thereafter, I started having mild but real contractions spaced about four minutes apart. I was terribly excited, but remembered all the reading I'd done for two years. I decided to work with the contractions for about an hour and a half and then see whether I could sleep through them. I could. It was delightful to wake the next morning knowing that my body could produce its own contractions. It didn't really matter that they hadn't gone anywhere. They were real and they were mine!

Saturday, March 13th

I have a rather empowering conversation with one of the midwives, in which I get her to admit that she was jumping the worry-gun a little soon. We move my appointment with the back-up doctor from Monday to Friday. I tell her I won't be pregnant by Monday anyway. (Ha ha ha.) That night, rather late, my vague contractions settled into ones that are coming very regularly at about 10 minutes apart and require me to concentrate through them. I was excited, but had a feeling this wasn't the Real Thing. So, I forced myself to go to sleep around 1 a.m. I woke up with a few of the contractions, but mostly I slept, and things fizzled out by midday Sunday.

Sunday, March 14th

My doula, Eileen, came over in the afternoon. She emphasized that I shouldn't get too excited—shouldn't try walking or anything else strenuous to get things moving faster. At this point, we were all still expecting that the baby would be born before my appointment with the midwives on Tuesday.

That night, the contractions got regular earlier (eight minutes apart) and I woke up with almost every single one. I drowsed in between and Todd and my mother took turns sitting up with me.

Monday, March 15th

I spent the better part of the day resting. I felt certain I'd be sprinting through the rest of the birth that night. I think I paid some bills and wrote email. I seem to recall needing to fling myself off the office chair and onto my knees, leaning on the bed for every contraction. They weren't particularly regular during the day, but they were continuing to be fairly intense.

Again that night, the contractions got regular and pretty intense. Still no "bloody show" [19] (mucus plug) and both Eileen and the midwives kept asking about that.

Tuesday, March 16th

The contractions stay intense all morning, but spread out to 10-20 minutes apart. Eileen comes with us to my appointment at the birth center. I'm about 2-3 cm, 50% effaced and the baby is at -1 station. We listen briefly to the heartbeat, but we don't do a Non-Stress Test (something I regret now). I tell everyone that I think the baby is posterior because I'm feeling nothing but hands and feet up front. In fact, my warning that a contraction is coming is that the baby starts flailing its arms and legs. Both the midwife and Eileen say there's just no way, since I'm not having *any* back labor whatsoever.

I think the midwife may have ascribed my slow-starting labor to VBAC "issues". Eileen was real big on saying that anything that was physically odd in labor had purely physical reasons. While I didn't believe her at first, it made more and more sense to me—especially because at that point I was SOOOO much further along than I ever got with my first birth. I figured that even if there had been any emotional issues holding me back, that I had to be past them already.

That night, the contractions did not settle into the tight rhythm that they had on previous evenings. I was beginning to lose track of the days—starting to feel like I was just going to spend the next month or two being almost in labor.

---

[19] *"Bloody show", or mucus plug, is a pinkish or bloody vaginal discharge, which many believe is an indicator that the first stage of labor is imminent.*

I really think I should emphasize that, although the contractions required concentration, and did in fact hurt—the whole thing was quite manageable. My husband was making sure I ate well and was drinking constantly. My mom was playing with my two-year-old. I was finding little projects to keep me occupied between contractions. The only thing that concerned me was keeping my strength and my spirits up for the Real Thing.

Wednesday, March 17th

About 2 a.m., I awaken terrified. It feels like I'm having one contraction on top of the other—maybe five peaks in a row. I just say, "Call Eileen" over and over. By the time Eileen gets to the house at about 3 a.m., I've settled back into my eight minutes apart routine. I feel a little silly for having called, but she is *so* much more helpful than my mother or Todd that I don't regret it. I try to sleep. Eileen stays awake and strokes my lower back with every single contraction, all night. The contractions seem stronger, and the back-stroking helps a *lot*.

The contractions continue all morning. By midday, we're sitting around wondering where to go from here. I'm feeling like I'm getting near the end of my tether. Eileen says it perfectly—that I'm doing beautifully, but I can't do another night like the last three and still have any energy left for the rest of the labor. She and Todd are plying me with blue & black cohosh. We finally decide to go for as much of a walk as I can stand. The contractions start coming four minutes apart. I hang on to Todd while Eileen strokes my back during each contraction and then we shuffle a few more steps.

Eileen starts talking about the possibility of convincing the midwives to break my waters. She feels I'm right on the edge and just need a little push over. She also says something about

153

wanting to see whether there's much meconium[20].

By this time, Caren (my friend who's going to be my son's caretaker while we're at the birth center) has arrived at the house. My contractions stay close and hard even after we're done walking. More time passes. I can only handle the pains when I'm standing and holding onto someone with Eileen stroking my back. I'm also getting this pinched nerve in my groin (another clue about head positioning).

I finally call the birth center. I talk for awhile with the midwife on call and she agrees to meet us at the center in an hour. We all get excited, pile everyone into three cars and head out.

When we get there, I am no more dilated or effaced than I was one and a half days prior and the baby is no lower. I work hard not to be disappointed. The midwife and student midwife hook me up for an NST. With the first contraction, we all instantly know that something's not right. The baby's heart rate remains unchanged *during* the contraction, but then drops off significantly as the contraction fades. We try some different positions, but get no change. The midwife (Pat) tells us we'll be heading for the hospital now. She tries to tell us that we aren't looking at an automatic c-section, but all I can think about is my first son's fetal distress. Everything just feels so horribly familiar. I keep thinking about all the work I've put into this birth so far—feeling like it was just a big waste of time.

---

[20] *"A dark green fecal material that accumulates in the fetal intestines and is discharged at or near the time of birth." Source: Dictionary.com Meconium present in the amniotic fluid may indicate fetal distress. If the baby inhales meconium, it can be dangerous. "Meconium aspiration is a leading cause of severe illness and death in the newborn." See:*
http://www.nlm.nih.gov/medlineplus/ency/article/001596.htm

Compounding the terror of another operation and another recovery is the fact that our insurance won't cover the doctor we're using and, therefore, might not cover any part of the hospital bill. Todd and I are having mild hysterics. I really let loose and just wept. Eileen said later that my emotional response was one of the things I'd been needing to do all week.

The hospital was extremely crowded that night. I thought I'd been put in a proper room on a proper bed. Todd told me later that it was actually a tiny exam room, and I was laboring on a gurney! I found out later that the Labor and Delivery nurse we dealt with that night had seen us coming in and insisted on being my nurse because she supported birth plans and midwives, etc. That was our one big stroke of luck. She also refused to take other patients so we had her undivided attention!

The doctor came in and checked me. During the car ride the baby had moved up to -3 station, but I was now 4 cm dilated! The midwives had given him a brief run-down of the last several days, and, as the monitor wasn't showing any fetal distress at all, he promptly broke my waters. Frankly, I was delighted. There was meconium in the fluid, but everyone was still talking vaginal birth, so I just settled into labor.

I was startled by how fast and furious the contractions started coming. Each one seemed too hard, and then it would pass and I'd feel great and perfectly capable of handling another. (What a thrill to labor without Pitocin!) Before long, I started getting transition symptoms. I refused to believe that I was at eight cm so quickly. It felt like it was only about two to three hours later. In fact, Eileen told me later, it was only a little over ONE hour later according to her notes. The nurse started scurrying to find a real delivery room at about the time that I lost patience with my husband. He's asthmatic and started having a bit of a coughing spell. I turned on him with, "Would you just *quit*! God! That's so distracting!!"

However, I was right, and I was only about six cm dilated, but almost completely effaced. (Another clue that the baby's head position was screwy!!) The baby's heart rate had started getting weird again and they kept me flopping from one side to the other to try to ease the pressure on the umbilical cord. Throughout all of this, I was feeling incredibly supported and completely buffered from typical hospital protocol. I had Todd, my doula, the midwife, student midwife and the great Labor and Delivery nurse surrounding me and giving me whatever I wanted.

Somewhere in there, I started getting pushing urges. They startled me and worried me. I just knew that I was still less than 8 cm (I was right) and I didn't want to get a cervical lip. I kept saying that to the midwife, and I think she kind of thought that was funny—that I was still so mentally focused that I was worrying about details like that. The urges were startling because they would come as a contraction was fading and they hit sort of like vomiting spasms. (Is this normal??) They weren't at all what I expected, but I recognized them immediately.

The midwives kept telling me that it was okay to go with the urges. I kept telling them that it *wasn't* okay yet. Something changed. Maybe my dilation was checked. They decided I'd been right not to push. I really think that breathing through the urge to push was the very hardest part of labor. The student midwife was holding my right hand. She had one hand on my chest and took every breath with me.

Sometime in here I was moved to a *real* Labor & Delivery room. Mostly the room annoyed me because it was big and lovely and I found that very distracting!

At some point, the doctor announced that I was "9 cm with an anterior lip."

I love this scene in my head because it shows the power of education and the beauty of a completely un-medicated labor. I was able to picture exactly what he was talking about and I remembered the remedy. I called down to him, "Can you hold it back and let me push past it?"

Being a good doctor, he responded, "That's what I'm doing."

About this time, we started pulling out all the stops and pushing like the dickens. I was not really understanding the urgency behind their demands to push so hard until someone strapped an oxygen mask over my face. They were obviously worried, but it was also this wonderfully supportive environment. I mean, I had a husband, a doula, two midwives, a nurse and a doctor telling me how strong I was and how great I was doing!

Then the doctor announces that the head is transverse and the baby is stuck at about 0 station. Again, I'm totally clear-headed. I ask whether he can adjust the head. He says he's trying to. A couple of pushes later, I hear the doctor say he'll be needing forceps. He calls in his partner for a consult. The other doctor watches me through a few contractions and agrees that forceps are appropriate.

Between contractions, I'm now saying, "Okay, so when do I get my drugs? Okay—I'm ready—what are you giving me??" I was kind of surprised that they chose to put an epidural in. I was expecting something more local. In retrospect, I'm pretty sure they did the epidural in case the forceps didn't work and we had to do a section. At the time, I had *no* idea how close I was to being sectioned.

So, after the next contraction, they flip me onto my side and give me the fastest epidural in the west. I'm amazed that *anyone* is capable of pushing a baby out with an epidural in. Even after all the pushing I'd just been doing, I had a very hard time figuring out what to do and when.

I notice Eileen taking flash photos of my crotch. I asked what was going on and someone told me that the head was out. I couldn't believe it! It was so unreal after all that work—and I really hadn't felt anything identifiable. I heard someone talking about the cord being tightly around the baby's neck. They cut the cord immediately, and, with the next contraction I felt the body slip out and that was a triumphant moment! My husband and I announced the sex. I told Todd to go talk to Eitan Lior while they were suctioning him (he was very floppy and not breathing yet). Todd said later that he was glad I'd announced the name, since he was so tired that he'd forgotten what name we'd agreed on!

The doc was stitching *forever*. He was very apologetic. He'd given me a "small" episiotomy and the forceps had given me a vaginal tear. He explained to me later that he had considered a c-section, but he'd realized that that would mean another 30 minutes to scrub in and get everything prepared and, with the forceps, he'd gotten the baby out in about 5-10 minutes. He also told me that he had manually checked my scar and everything was fine internally. I'm glad I had the epidural during that little procedure. It was that one thing that I disagreed with him about, but it just didn't matter so much after all the drama of getting the baby out.

Eitan was born at 6:53 a.m. on Thursday, March 18th. By 6:00 that evening, we'd been cleared for discharge and I went home with all my boys—sore but triumphant.

Over the next few days all four midwives from the birth center phoned to see whether I was disappointed about how the birth had turned out. I kept laughing at them. Seems they

> *I have zero problem with medical technology being used when it is absolutely necessary.*

get lots of people with very fixed ideas of what their births should look like—people who get pissed off if they don't have their perfect, candle-lit water-births. I told them I was thrilled! I have zero problem with medical technology being used when it is absolutely necessary. And the whole process had proven that I was right to go with the midwives and doctor who seemed the best fit, in spite of the fact that my insurance didn't cover anything except the hospital stay.

There are two themes to this story: The baby's head position makes all the difference in the world; and so does having the right medical/support team.

Shortly after the birth, I'd been saying to people that I'd give birth again in a heartbeat. Unfortunately, I couldn't stand the thought of more children! I was totally overwhelmed by diapers and crying and sleep deprivation (and that was just the two-year-old!)

Wendy Bat-Sarah is mama to Avi (born 10/25/96 by c-section for fetal distress) and Eitan (born 3/18/99 by VBAC with forceps-assist).

18. I Will Definitely Do It Again!
by Franny Meritt

To prepare for this birth, I gathered some very special Christian women around me for a Blessing God's Way. This is a selection that I have written about in Abby's baby book

Our midwife started off by reading Genesis 3:16-17.

> [16] *To the woman He said: "I will greatly multiply your sorrow and your conception; In **pain** you shall bring forth children; Your desire shall be for your husband, And he shall rule over you."*

> [17] *Then to Adam He said, "Because you have heeded the voice of your wife, and have eaten from the tree of which I commanded you, saying, 'You shall not eat of it': "Cursed is the ground for your sake; In **toil** you shall eat of it all the days of your life.*

(Genesis 3:16-17 CIV)

The sad thing about this passage is that, over the years, it has been mistranslated. Both of the bold/underlined words are the same word, etsev. It means hard work and that is what labor is, hard work, just like working in the garden. I've worked in the garden all summer to have fresh food to eat to help you grow healthy and to prepare me for the hard work of your birth.

At 10 days past my due date, I was miserable and called my midwife for help. This pregnancy lasted more than two weeks longer than my first, and six weeks longer than my second. I felt like I was going to be pregnant forever. My midwife recommended that I see the chiropractor and get a massage. I chose the latter and by evening (Wednesday) contractions had started. I went about my normal activities, fixed supper, went to church, bathed the kids, put them to bed, and went for a walk. Contractions were regular, but not very strong (more like annoying). Thursday morning, we were supposed to drive an hour away to see the midwife. I didn't think I could handle being in the car that long so I told her to head our way. I napped and felt like they were fading away, and was nearly resigned to the fact that it just wasn't time yet.

A few days earlier, I went into work for a bridal shower and one of my co-workers, an Ob/Gyn Nurse Practitioner, said I should just go to the hospital and have another cesarean since I was so far over my due date. I had a lot of mental work to do to get over that.

Our midwife arrived at 3:00 p.m. and I told her what I was thinking/feeling. She helped me get rid of that baggage. Within a half hour, my water broke.

I knew mentally I would have a lot of work to do. The following verses were the focus of my Blessing God's Way. It took a lot of work to redirect my focus away from the discomfort and toward God's glory. I think eventually I just learned that, though labor was very intense, it would end soon and I needed that trial to help prepare me to parent this new life.

6Don't worry about anything; instead, pray about everything. Tell God what you need, and thank him for all he has done. If you do this, you will experience God's peace, which is far more wonderful than the human mind can understand. His peace will guard your hearts and minds as you live in Christ Jesus.

8And now, dear brothers and sisters, let me say one more thing as I close this letter. Fix your thoughts on what is true and honorable and right. Think about things that are pure and lovely and admirable. Think about things that are excellent and worthy of praise.

(Philippians 4:6-8 CIV)

By 5:00 p.m., my doula and our friends who were coming to help watch our older two kids were present and I was starting to get uncomfortable. Around 7:00 p.m., I was four cm (the first time my midwife had ever examined me). I got in the tub (borrowed a spa in a box from a friend) and got hot, then had to get out to cool off.

I had just attended a Michel Odent conference and had his words in my head. If a woman gets in the tub at 4:00 and makes no rapid progress after two hours, he recommended a cesarean. I kept thinking that I didn't have the urge to push, so had I made progress?

After dark (9ish?), I got back in the tub and was very cold. My husband found a space heater and was holding it on me next to the tub and jokingly went "oops" faking dropping it into the tub. After that, it took me over an hour to get back into a regular pattern. I was shivering constantly, and eventually had to get into the shower to get warmed back up. My midwife thought my shivering was also due to lack of energy/calories. She and my doula encouraged me to drink some really salty, hot broth.

By 11:00 p.m., I was loud and hurting. They also worked to get me to eat a peanut butter and jelly sandwich, and to drink some juice. Peanut butter is NOT easy to get down with 'labor mouth'. I was all over the place, constantly changing positions. I remember feeling best in a forward leaning position. I starting pushing around midnight, although my midwife said I wasn't *really pushing* until about 1:00 or so.

I started in the tub at first, but kept a rim of cervix and got out to the birth stool so the midwife could help hold it while I pushed. While on the birth stool, I remember saying, "I give up. Take me to the hospital, Help me." And, they gave me some homeopathy.

The midwife said, "Finally, it's time to have a baby!" They told me it wouldn't be long and I got back in the tub.

The midwife said I have 'a large perineum' and so it felt like crowning took FOREVER. I remembered what it was like with Daniel, my first child, and I realized that I never got to the point where I could push past the pain and make progress. I finally figured out how to push this time, but the pushing into the pain to make progress, then the contraction ending and feeling the baby slide back up and knowing I'd have to push back through that pain again with the next contraction, was nearly overwhelming.

I was on my knees in the tub, resting my head on the side of the tub. Aryn put his arm along the back of the tub so I could rest my head and I accidentally bit him. I didn't even realize I was doing it until he flinched.

I got to the point where I felt like my urethra was going to explode and I reached down to support my labia and felt her head. It didn't take long from that point. It was so empowering to realize how close I really was.

Once her head was out, her body followed quickly. The midwife just allowed the water to catch her. When she was out, I flipped over and reached for her. Within a few seconds, I was pulling her up so I could see her, unlooped two nuchal cords and brought her out of the water to my chest. She opened her eyes and looked at me and started to whimper. No lusty, painful scream, but more like, "Wait a second, what just happened?"

163

I felt between her legs and discovered she was a girl, but waited until our son came into the room to lift her out of the water for him to see and announce. I was convinced I was having a boy because my pregnancy was so much like it was with Daniel. Instead, I have a little girl that looks just like her big brother.

The placenta came about 15 minutes after her birth and I was out of the tub 30 minutes after her birth. We left the cord attached for about two hours. At that point, we were able to cut without clamping and it fell off when she was 4 days old. I had a small 'scuff', but nothing worth suturing. My midwife had an herbal bath to soak in with Abby and it felt wonderful. I had to learn the hard way to strain out the herbs though. They clogged the tub. Abby nursed very well and my milk was in within about 24 hours. She never lost weight. She was 8 lbs, 5 oz at birth, at 2:04 a.m. Friday, October 14th and was 8 lbs, 9 oz on Monday evening. Abigail has been a joy, a wonderful baby. I will definitely do it again!!!

This was an editorial (see next chapter) I sent to our local newspaper after my daughter's birth, explaining my decision and outcome in relation to the release of 2004 c-section rates. Several of the OB's in our area were really ticked when they found out I was the Childbirth Educator at the local Medicaid clinic. Our Medical Director wanted me to assure him that I was not teaching or encouraging home birth in my class. I replied that I simply told my story and that I did not believe that home birth was an option for our clients for two reasons...they can't afford the out of pocket expense of home birth and local doctors refuse to provide back up. When patients ask, I simply inform them that home birth is legal, and the experts in home birth are not, but they do exist.

I Chose Not to Become a Statistic

by Franny Meritt

For the Journal and Courier

http://www.lafayettejc.com/apps/pbcs.dll/article?AID=/20051121/OPIN
ION03/511210303/1144/OPINION

The results are in and 2004 saw another increase in surgical birth rates -- 29.1 percent of women delivered their babies by cesarean last year, according to a National Center for Health Statistics report released last week.

Some doctors cited the reason for the increase was that more women are having elective cesareans, but keep in mind that "elective" does not mean that it was the woman's choice.

Earlier this year, when we discovered we were expecting our third baby, I visited my Ob/Gyn to begin prenatal care. I was informed that we would be forced to have a cesarean if our baby was born at their hospital simply because I had a cesarean with my second child (because she was in a transverse lie at 36 weeks after spontaneous rupture of membranes).

The cesarean rate has increased astronomically in the past 30 years: 5.5 percent in 1970, 16.5 percent in 1980, and 22.7 percent in 2000. The World Health Organization states that the cesarean rate should be 10 percent to 15 percent. Our bodies have not changed in 30 years, but medical management has. Although some babies have been saved by surgical delivery, a look at maternal and infant mortality rates show that nearly 30 countries lose fewer moms and babies than the United States and most of those countries have lower cesarean rates.

Having a vaginal birth after cesarean (VBAC) carries nearly half the potential complications than repeat surgery. Due to a 0.5 percent to 1 percent risk of uterine rupture, The American College of Obstetricians and Gynecologists has put very strict guidelines on VBAC, stating that the doctor and operating team need to be immediately available.

American Academy of Family Physicians guidelines noted that there are other problems that occur more often, and they found no evidence suggesting better VBAC outcomes based on the availability of resources. American Academy of Family Physicians went on to state that policies for VBAC "appear to be based on malpractice concerns rather than on available statistical and scientific evidence."

So, how'd I do it? I hired a midwife and kept my OB/GYN as backup. I found a doula—someone trained to provide emotional and physical support during labor (http://www.lafayettedoulas.com) — and obtained a portable hot tub for pain relief. I ate well and read to educate myself. When labor started, my midwife came to me, and my daughter was safely born at home in water. (See http://www.babiesonline.com/babies/a/abbyrae).

I'll do it again with my next baby. As long as doctors and hospitals do not allow alternatives, such as midwives, birthing centers and natural options for pain relief, more informed women who want to be able to make their own decisions will join me.

Franny Meritt is a pastor's wife, mother of three, RN and childbirth educator at a Community Health Clinic. Franny enjoys gardening and sewing and is in the process of starting a Christ Centered Childbirth Class.

19. Our Bodies Will Do Anything to Protect Our Babies
by Lauren Cooper

My first cesarean was planned and necessary due to a birth defect my daughter had—gastroschesis. When I became pregnant with my second daughter, I went back and forth with the idea of VBAC. Once I decided to VBAC, I decided to have a natural, intervention-free birth to ensure my baby's safety and my success. I did the research. I threw out my copy of <u>What to Expect When You're Expecting</u>, and got the REAL birth books, I hired a doula, I wrote a birth plan, and I made sure my doctor was on board with me. I even played with the idea of home birth, but (unfortunately) I let my fears of the "what ifs" and the unknown guide me to the (wrong) decision of staying with planning a hospital birth. I thought that I had the proper knowledge, support, and strength to be able to advocate for myself and get the birth that I wanted, and knew I could have.

I went into labor after my doctor stripped my membranes without my knowledge or consent. When I showed up at the hospital around 2 a.m., after already having been in labor at my home for almost an entire day beforehand, they conveniently could not find my birth plan that I had just recently ensured that they had on file. I had a copy of my birth plan that had been signed by my regular OB with me and I gave it to the staff, but it didn't matter. Even though I gave them the copy of my birth plan that was signed saying that I was refusing routine things such as the IV, continuous monitoring, and wearing their hospital gowns, among other things, I still had to fight these things away.

When I arrived at the hospital the nurse checked me and told me I was 4 cm. I continued to labor, mostly in the shower, but occasionally tried other things like walking the halls, bouncing on the birth ball, and laboring on all fours. A few hours after arriving at the hospital, a different doctor—not my regular OB—came on call, checked me and told me that I was *still* at 4 cm. He told me I could continue as I was, which obviously wasn't getting me anywhere (his words), I could be augmented with having my waters broken and taking Pitocin, or I could just go on in for the repeat cesarean. I told him that I chose to continue to labor as I was seeing as my baby and I were doing just fine. He left and soon returned, telling me that I had to get in bed and be hooked up to continuous monitoring. When I asked him why, he told me it was simply because I was going for a VBAC. I asked him if there was reason for concern, and he told me yes, that because I was VBAC, my uterus could explode and my baby and I could die. I asked if my baby and I were currently showing any signs of distress and he said no, so I reminded him that my regular OB had signed my birth plan saying that just intermittent monitoring was fine and that I'd like to just continue as I am. He made me sign a waiver clearly stating that I understood that without the continuous monitoring, I know that my uterus could explode and my baby and I could die (even though this can very well happen with the monitoring, anyway).

I continued to labor and he checked me a few more times throughout the afternoon, each time proclaiming, "You're *still* at 4 cm and your baby isn't engaged, no progress what-so-ever." Each time he reminded me of my options—stay as I was, which was getting me nowhere, get augmented with Artificial Rupture of the Membranes (AROM), Pitocin, and continuous monitoring, or just go on ahead with the repeat cesarean.

A little after 4 p.m. that afternoon, I finally gave in to the pressures to have my waters broken since I was being told that

I hadn't progressed at all in the 14 hours I'd been there and I continued to labor in the shower. By the time 6 p.m. hit, my contractions were coming every 2 minutes and often closer, one right after the other, each lasting well over a minute long. I did nothing but moan during the contractions while I squatted in the shower. I did this for a few hours until I started to feel pressure in my bottom. It wasn't this big huge urge to push, but it was definitely pressure, I could feel her moving down. I wanted to be checked. I wanted that reassurance because I KNEW I had made progress, I could just feel it.

Upon being checked, he told me that I was wrong, my baby was not engaged (of course, this is what gravity does when you throw a woman flat on her back and check for dilation) and I was *still* only 4 cm. He again told me my options, while stating that it was getting late and that he and the anesthesiologist were going home soon, and that if at some point during the night my baby or I did need a cesarean, no one would be immediately available to perform one and save us.

We asked him to leave the room while my husband, my doula and I discussed what to do. In other words, I sat there and cried and cried, tired and in so much pain, as my husband looked on, crying as well. My doula said that, at this point, another cesarean probably wasn't a bad idea since I was not progressing on my own and agreeing to Pitocin could be very dangerous to me and to my baby because I had a scarred uterus. I died inside at that moment, knowing that I had no support left. I told the doctor we'd go ahead with another cesarean, all the while saying that if I had just progressed past 4 cm that I'd have the strength to continue on and keep trying. After 42 hours of labor, at 10:21 that night, my baby girl was extracted from me, and funny thing, even though she supposedly wasn't engaged, she had an awfully molded head.

I sort of denied how I really felt about the entire thing during my painful yet "normal" physical recovery. I started having nightmares about the entire ordeal (the cesarean and the treatment I received, not the labor itself) while still in the hospital, but I tried to dismiss them and just focus on my new little baby.

A few months passed and, after some resistance from the hospital, my records that I requested were finally sent to me. There in the records was very clearly written that I had in fact been 5-6 cm dilated and that I did not officially stall until he placed that seed of doubt in my mind. When I found out I had been going through this awful emotional roller coaster for months completely unnecessarily, this is when the Post Traumatic Stress Disorder really kicked in full force. The nightmares persisted, the anxiety and panic attacks threatened me every day, and the thoughts about it are with me every waking moment of every day. Even the nurses' notes clearly proclaimed that I was 5-6 cm; the same nurses that were there when he checked me and heard him tell me I was 4 cm the entire time wrote down that I had been told I was 5-6 cm. The same nurse that went out and informed my entire family in the waiting room that I was finally giving in and having the repeat cesarean because I have been stuck at 4 cm for so long had "5-6 cm" clearly written in her records as well. There is no way this was simply a miscommunication or that I misheard anything. Yes, I was tired and in a lot of pain, but my husband, my doula, and my entire family waiting in the waiting room all heard the same thing—I was told I was only 4 cm the entire time.

The doctor's intentions may not necessarily have been to make me end in a cesarean, but they most certainly were to gain control of me and my labor. Our bodies are amazing things and will do anything to protect our babies. It's instinctive for a mother's body to keep the baby inside where it is safe, away from any threats the mother is feeling when in labor, which is what my body was doing. I was not feeling safe or supported in that environment, and his lies are what placed that seed of doubt in my mind, making my progression seemingly stall. Eleven months after the fact and I still can't get it all out of my head for more than a few seconds at a time. It's consumed me, it's become who I am, it has cost me so much already, and it will continue to make me miss out on so many things for the rest of my life.

I've tried to do everything to stop this sorry excuse of a doctor and those awful nurses who heard him lying to me from doing this to others, but to no avail. I've contacted lawyers, written letters to the hospital, sent in formal complaints to the State Department of Health, sent story submissions into local newspapers and television stations, but I've gotten nowhere with all of these things. In the eyes of the law, my baby and I were not harmed (ha!) by this since we are alive and have no permanent damage (again, ha!). There is nothing I can legally do. The hospital has basically ignored my concerns, and has even stopped providing me with any more of my records or explanations, stating that, because of the investigation that my complaints launched by the State Department of Health, they are no longer comfortable providing me with any more of (my own) records or explanations thereof. The State Department of Health basically said that it is a "He said, she said" thing that they can't prove one way or the other, so they can't (won't) do anything about it. Television stations and newspapers tell me that they don't want to get in the middle of it and, without anything concrete, they can't do a story on it. So, I've had to rely on word of mouth to try and save others from going through the hell that I live with each day now.

Since I've been trying to get the word out locally, I've had a number of other women, mostly young adults like myself, contact me about their similar run-ins with this same doctor and

> *Women don't need to be saved from birth—they need to be saved from the birth rape that is being done to them in western medicine's mismanagement of birth.*

hospital, and I'm so saddened and sickened by this. He's done this to so many women before who didn't even know they had a choice or could do anything about it. He did it to me and he'll continue to do it to others. And it's not just him; it's everywhere in medicalized birth today, and it's a very scary and sad thing to have such a beautiful, normal, natural process turned into something medicalized, and treated like a sickness that the average woman, who is not on the godly level of the almighty doctor, is treated as if she's not capable of doing without intervention or a doctor there to save her from birth. Women don't need to be saved from birth—they need to be saved from the birth rape that is being done to them in western medicine's mismanagement of birth.

We do plan on having more children and, when we do, we are happily planning a beautiful, peaceful, natural home birth so that our baby will be safely welcomed into loving, trustworthy hands. But it's never going to be easy—I'll always have these fears and doubts now. I'm sure everyone does, but mine feel magnified, and I'm really hoping that some day I will find peace and meaning in all of this. Until then, I just feel so trapped, so consumed by this. I don't wish this on anyone.

Lauren Cooper, a stay at home mom to her two daughters Mykaylah and Lydia, is currently planning with her husband Todd on trying to conceive another child, their HBA2C-hopeful baby. She has become active in spreading knowledge of the birthing rights of women and babies and encourages all women who are pregnant or planning on becoming pregnant to contact ICAN (http://www.ican-online.org) and the Trust Birth Initiative (http://www.trustbirth.org) to receive valuable information and support.

20. Stuck at 4 cm...
by Kathleen F.

I would love to blame everyone and everything present in the delivery room on March 4, 2003 for my cesarean section—the doctors, the nurses, my husband, the fetal monitor, the IV, the epidural, and, most especially, me. However, if I blame all of those people and all of those things for the failure of my first attempt at a vaginal birth, then I could not very well give those same people and that same technology the credit they deserve for the success of my second attempt at a vaginal birth.

My first daughter, Bridget, was delivered via c-section at 6:52 p.m. on March 4th, after being induced 23 hours earlier. My daughter was and is perfectly healthy; she was a big baby and I only progressed to four centimeters after all that labor. She weighed nine pounds, one ounce, and had a head full of curly black hair and lungs that carried her scream throughout the entire hospital.

When I got pregnant with Ivy, my second daughter, in March of 2005, I decided that everything would be different this time. No doctors, no nurses, no monitors, no hospital. I was going to have a home birth with a midwife and a doula. This birth would be in a birthing pool, no less, with dimmed lights, soothing music and my rapturous cries as I birthed my baby vaginally. To ensure success, I did everything different during my pregnancy with Ivy. I did not have any prenatal testing done. I only went to the obstetrician to secure his approval to serve as a backup in case of transfer, and I even gained fifteen pounds less than I did with Bridget. Since I was induced with Bridget two days after my due date, I was prepared to wait on Ivy.

Six days after December 23, my due date, I went into labor, and Ivy was born three days later, on New Year's Day. That's right, three days of labor before my eight pound, seven ounce caterwauling daughter was born, with a head full of straight brown hair and lungs just like her sister.

However, Ivy's birth was nothing like I had envisioned for myself during the many months of my pregnancy. She was born in a hospital, birthed through my vagina, and caught by a doctor in a harshly-lit delivery room, with monitors attached to both of us, an epidural in my spine and an IV in my arm. What went wrong? Well, nothing, I would argue, since I did successfully birth an incredibly healthy baby. What changed my plans so drastically? I transferred to the hospital after three exhausting, exhilarating days of labor due to maternal exhaustion.

I woke up in labor on Thursday, December 29th. The contractions were light enough that I continued with my daily activities, although I was already pretty tired from not resting well and also taking care of a toddler full-time. I called my doula and gave her a heads up that I might need her soon, and she talked me though the things to look for and reminded me of positions to try. Most of all, she just encouraged me to stay focused and that everything would be all right. Thursday night was rough, with my contractions coming closer together and much harder, although there was no pattern to them at all. I could not sleep through them, although I did sleep in between them. I got up Friday, absolutely worn out, but determined to keep going. Little did I know that the exhaustion I was feeling would be nothing compared to the exhaustion that would drive me to the hospital late Saturday night.

I called my doula again Friday morning and told her what was happening. She suggested a warm bath and said she'd be there after lunch. I had contractions every three to five minutes, sometimes six minutes apart, all day. They were strong contractions, too strong for me to move around while they were happening, although I could talk through some of them and not through others. The contractions were very inconsistent. When my doula arrived, she began to time them and was confused by their irregularity. I was terrified that I wasn't really in labor and that possibly these pains would go away with nightfall. She reassured me that I was truly in labor and that women sometimes labor differently.

My doula offered to check my cervix, and I agreed, mainly because I was getting desperate at that point and needed to know that I was truly in labor. I had had some bloody show (mucus plug), but not a big gloppy mess that I hoped for, so dilation would really indicate whether I was in true labor or not.

She checked me around 6:00 p.m. on Friday night, and I was at four centimeters. Ah, the cursed number four, that most reviled of all numbers that had won me a C-section the first time. However, she did not allow me to get discouraged by not being any further along than four. She declared that the baby was asynclitic (tilted to one side), and had me labor on my side for a while to try to get her to turn her head straight and apply more pressure to my cervix. I hurt laboring on my side; I hurt laboring standing, sitting, leaning, walking. I just plain old hurt. My contractions were still irregular, although they were much stronger and much closer together.

We called the midwife around 11:00 p.m. Friday night and told her to come on; my doula was fairly certain that my contractions would continue to come quicker and closer together, and we both needed more support. I had been in labor for over forty hours by now, and my doula and my husband needed a break as well. The midwife lived almost two hours away, so by the time she got her things together and got here, it was around 2:00 a.m.. I was very stressed by this point, since I had not prepared myself to labor this long.

I knew I would have a long labor, since I had labored with Bridget for 23 hours before my c-section. Somehow, I guess I just didn't think that my body would repeat those same mistakes again. When the midwife got to my house, she checked me and pronounced that I was still at four centimeters. I almost completely gave up at that point. I was so angry at my lack of progression, and about her casual attitude towards it, that I wanted to scream and cry and collapse and never, ever have the baby. I wanted my labor to stop and the baby to just stay inside forever.

The midwife made some suggestions that seemed ridiculous at the time, although in retrospect they were very wise. She and the doula gave me a full-body massage to relax me. At first, I really resisted their touch and tensed up. My tension only made the contractions hurt worse, and did nothing for my state of mind. Those two women persisted, though, and I relaxed. After that massage, the rest of my labor until Ivy was born at 2:57 a.m. on Sunday, January 1, is pretty much a blur. I had always read about women in labor entering an altered state of conscience, but I didn't think that would happen to me. I try to always be in control, on top of things, and I am usually unwilling to let events unfold around me. But after the midwife said I was still at four centimeters, I think I just shut down.

My mother came to town early Saturday morning from her house, which is three hours away, with the intention of taking Bridget with her to a hotel. However, my in-laws, who also live three hours away, showed up shortly afterward and took Bridget with them. Although she had originally had no intention of staying while I labored, she quickly changed her mind when I asked her to stay. Seeing me, she said later, changed her entire attitude about a laboring woman. She told me that she had never known that someone could be as strong as I was, and that I was so willing to just let go and follow my body. I am glad that she saw some nobility in my agony, since at the time I felt nothing but misery.

At five o'clock that afternoon, I finally went into transition. Sixty hours after my labor began, I was finally at ten centimeters, throwing up, and shaking. Then my water broke, which was fairly uneventful, since I was heaving into a trashcan at the time. Once I got to ten centimeters, I vaguely remember being very impressed with myself. My c-section with Bridget had been deemed medically necessary for failure to progress. Well, I suppose it was really failure to wait, since it took me so long to finally get to ten centimeters.

I moved to the bathtub shortly after my water broke, because I was having some bizarre and incredibly painful sensations in my perineal area, which the midwife attributed to a desire to push. Well, it wasn't a desire to push; it turned out later that it was the back of Ivy's big head pushing down on my internal hemorrhoids, causing the most horrendous pain that I can imagine. I pushed anyway, for four hours, in innumerable positions, with little progress.

At 10:30 p.m., I snapped. I stood up, and said in a very calm voice, "I am going to the hospital. James, you are going to take me. Mother, you are coming with us. Let's go. Now."

I had had enough. I had been eating and drinking during labor, but since I hit transition and threw it all up, I felt drained and empty, far emptier than I had in the previous three days. I knew something was wrong, I just didn't know what. The midwife checked the baby's heart tones one last time and said she was fine, no decelerating, and asked if I wanted to try another position to get her to move a little in my pelvis and rotate. I replied that there was nothing she or anyone else could do to

177

make me try one more position, and that I was going to the hospital.

After an almost-comical trip to the hospital, with my husband driving way too fast and me screaming as we hit every bump and divot in the road, we arrived around 11:15 p.m.. I was whisked to a room, screaming the whole way, plopped in a bed and given an IV. I started to feel better, although the contractions were right on top of each other. I was in agony, but the nurse was wonderful, coaching me quietly and encouraging me every single minute.

She literally did not stop talking to me or touching my leg or arm for the almost hour wait I had until the doctor finally arrived. He took one look at me and ordered an epidural; I begged for a c-section. I actually looked him in the eye and said, "Section me. Please."

He said no, let's wait for the epidural and then see what's going on. After the epidural, he reached in, felt the cranial sutures on Ivy's head, and declared that she was indeed asynclitic, and posterior as well. With one fluid movement, he reached in, turned her, and declared that we had merely to wait and she would be born.

After two more hours of pushing, Ivy Ruedell was finally born.

Kathleen and James live in Mississippi and are the proud parents of Bridget, 3, and Ivy, 4 months. Kathleen is a full-time stay at home mom, although she occasionally teaches a college English course at night at the local university. James is a computer programmer at one of the nation's largest telecommunications companies.

21. Hoping for a Better VBAC Next Time...
by Emilie

My husband, an infantry soldier in the Army, was deployed for the last six months of my pregnancy with our first child, Gavin Lee. I decided to go home and be with our families during his deployment, and so I had seen a civilian OB during my whole pregnancy. He came home September 27th, 2002 and was able to start a 2-week leave around the beginning of October. We were posted in Fort Benning, Georgia but, during his leave, we came home to Michigan with all intentions of bringing back our little boy bundle that was due October 27th.

My OB decided to give me a late trimester ultrasound because she was not sure of our son's size. She told me that he was going to be 11-12 lbs, and she recommended that I deliver him via c-section. I was extremely reluctant and disappointed, but she was pretty insistent. In addition, my husband's leave was almost over and he was worried that he would not be able to see the birth of our son, so he ended up persuading me to have a c-section.

On October 18th, my beautiful, big eyed, perfect baby boy came into the world screaming before they even pulled him out of my womb. I laughed so hard and cried at the same time. My husband laughed and had tears in his eyes. Gavin was 8 pounds, 8ounces.

I had a terrible, long recovery. It took me months to feel like myself again. I got an infection in my incision, fluid built up and it had to be reopened. It took a very long time to heal. I struggled with postpartum exhaustion and depression and I was not even able to enjoy my brand new baby. I just remember crying a lot.

When Gavin was about 16 months old, we learned that I was pregnant again. My husband had just recently returned home from Iraq and we were on our way to Fort Wainwright, Alaska. I was absolutely determined to do a VBAC. Having another c-section was just not an option to me. I wanted to deliver my baby the "natural" way.

I know I am extremely lucky to have had such a supportive healthcare team at the military hospital where we were posted. It seemed like having another c-section was not an option to them either. They encouraged me throughout my whole pregnancy, and I only had to sign one form!! I dragged my husband to four weeks of childbirth classes and really concentrated on what I would do to have a drug-free, as-natural-as-can-be vaginal birth. I read all of the books, I did all of the research, and I believed in my heart that this birth would be the one I wanted.

My son was due September 27, 2004. On October 10th, he was still having a grand old time camping out and enjoying life in mom's belly. I, however, was not enjoying myself and I was so extremely desperate to give birth I was not tolerable to my poor husband, or anyone else who was in contact with me. My midwife did an ultrasound and told me that, even though baby was fine, the placenta was getting old, and she would be more comfortable if I was induced the following week. She did strip my membranes for the third time in a row and told me to go home, rock on the birthing ball, walk, relax, and have lots of sex. Some of these things were done much easier, and with much less complaining from my husband than other things. She wished me luck, and told me she hoped I would go into labor that weekend.

October 13th, I went into the hospital at 6:30 a.m. to be induced. I was set up with an IV and the extremely fashionable, yet not quite comfortable monitors, and then just waited for the midwife to show up. She got there around 8:00 a.m., and started me on Pitocin. I didn't really get any contractions for a good hour or so, but when they finally did start, they were very strong and very close together. I hung in there until about 11:30 a.m. Doing my breathing, squeezing my husbands hand, concentrating on my son's picture, etc., I was starting to get pretty panicky and feeling like there was no way I could do this anymore when my blood pressure started to shoot up. Then, the baby's heartbeat started dipping to an unsafe level during my contractions. I was having piggyback contractions that were lasting 90 seconds, and about 10-15 seconds apart because of the Pitocin. The contractions were squeezing the baby for too long and too hard and that's why his heartbeat was dipping. My blood pressure was shooting up because of how painful and intense they were.

The nurse rushed in, turned me on my left side, and put an oxygen mask on me. The midwife came in within a few seconds afterwards, turned down the Pitocin, and told me she thought I would do much better with an epidural. At that time, I don't think any words could have been much sweeter to me. I agreed, very willingly, and the anesthesiologist came in about 45 minutes later to start my push button epidural. Around 12:30 p.m. I was feeling so much better, and really was thinking that this was the way to go.

From 12:30 p.m. to around 11:00 p.m. things went pretty much uneventfully. I was very impressed every time the monitor would show I was having a contraction and the nurse said that I had dilated, and yet I didn't feel a blessed thing. I watched T.V., chatted with my hubby, took a nap, and just waited.

At around 11:00 p.m. my nurse came in and told me I was 10 centimeters and that I could start pushing. I was so excited and pushed with all of my might and heart. After about an hour and a half of this, I was feeling more irritated than excited and I was getting tired of the whole process. One thing that did not help was that I had been so intent on pushing that I was not pushing the button for my epidural, and let myself get in quite a bit of pain before I noticed.

Very, very quickly, around 12:30 a.m., I started to have some pretty unbearable pain and I was so incredibly nauseous. I could not quit chomping on those ice chips. I had to have them in my mouth all of the time or else I knew I was going to be pushing and puking at the same time. I was not really ready to have that much fun yet.

Around 1:30 a.m., I decided that I was done and I seemed to take things very personally. One thing that I remember quite clearly is my husband leaning on the safety rail on the edge of the bed, just watching me. I looked at him and snapped, "Stop looking at me!" He was so sweet and did all of the good coaching things that he was taught in our childbirth classes. It really infuriated me, however, that he was insisting that I push for 10 of his seconds, when I wanted to push for 10 of my seconds, and I thought I, the one trying to push the baseball out of a straw, probably knew better than him, the one sitting there in no pain. His voice was grating on my nerves to an intolerable level and I finally just told him to please, please, just quit talking. Period. Everything we learned in our childbirth classes pretty much all went out the window.

By this time, my midwife had gone off shift and I had an OB that I had only seen once through my pregnancy taking care of me. My baby had a very large head and quite a cone on top that he thought was due to me pushing for so long. He was very encouraging and told me that he knew I could do this. He really did not want to have to do a c-section on me and he knew that I did not want that either. I was feeling the full effects of my contractions, and the Pitocin, and I have never known such pain in my entire life. It was unreal. I was panicking, not keeping it together or being rational in the very least. My teeth were chattering and I was shaking violently. The same anesthesiologist was called in and he gave me a bolus of pain medication but, by this time, there was just no helping or turning around.

At around 2:00 a.m., I had been pushing for three hours and was so exhausted and weak. I was making no progress, the baby was still high, and the OB decided to use forceps. He waited through two contractions, and than one more because I begged him to, and than he finally inserted them. If I thought I was in pain before, then I was sadly mistaken. The pressure was almost unbearable and I remember just starting to scream. At the time, it seemed as though the nurses and the doctor were being very mean to me. They kept telling me in no uncertain terms to quit screaming and push. Now I know they were trying to get me to calm down and concentrate on pushing, to assist the OB since my baby was so high. A nurse and my husband grabbed my hands and I did NOT want to be touched. They let go very quickly, probably because I shouted at them to not touch me. They put oxygen on me and my husband would spoon in ice chips one right after the other, I was still extremely nauseous.

Five full contractions later, my second baby boy, Nathan Levi, finally came into this world. He was 9 pounds, 1 ounce. It was all so surreal. I lay back with almost no emotions at all like I had with Gavin. My husband, the nurses, the OB, and the anesthesiologist were all so happy and excited. Some of them were laughing and my husband and the anesthesiologist had tears in their eyes. I felt almost emotionless. I was the only one not laughing or crying or excited. I was exhausted and could not keep my eyes open. Also, my nausea had climaxed and I threw up while they were still drying my son off. I had a second degree tear that the OB sewed up. Immediately after delivering the placenta, my nurse gave me a shot of Phenergan to take away my nausea and I almost instantly drifted off into sleep, without holding my baby son even once.

About five hours later, I woke up and the nurse brought him in so that I could finally meet him, breastfeed, and cuddle with him. I think an awful birthing experience, exhaustion, and disappointment prevented me from really bonding with him until I got home. I was, and still am, disappointed with everything that went wrong with my birthing experience. It was not how I wanted it to be.

I am now pregnant with our third little boy and planning another VBAC. Even though I had a better birth with my c-section, I had so many complications during the recovery that it took me months before I felt back to myself again. With my VBAC, I was sore for several weeks, but other than that the recovery was vastly better than the one with my c-section. There are two things I will do differently this time around. The first is I will not be induced unless absolutely medically necessary, I really feel it contributed to one complication after another, and that I would have had a much better experience had I not been induced. The second is that I am not expecting this birth to go any certain way at all. All I can do is hope that the saying "third time is a charm" is true.

Emilie is 23 years old and married to her high school sweetheart, Nathan. Her husband recently got out of the army. They have two naughty but charming little boys, and their third boy is due July 1st, 2006. Emilie graduated from nursing school in December of 2005 and plans to work in a VA hospital after the baby is born.

22. The Happiest Mom
with a Sore Bottom in Town
by J.P.

My introduction to childbirth was at my first job as a nurse in the labor and delivery unit at a community hospital. I developed skills in supporting women who desired natural and un-medicated childbirth. Working during the night shift afforded me the opportunity to spend many hours with laboring women without interruption by physicians who generally preferred to sleep until the mother was ready to deliver. I preferred working with women who presented in spontaneous labor to the induced and highly managed labor. Of course, when I had to circulate the Operating Room for a woman needing a cesarean, I would think to myself, "I hope that never happens to me! I wouldn't want to be cut open like that." As nurses we would try very hard to keep our patients out of the operating room, usually advocating for a little more time for a mom going slowly or encouraging a mother to change positions often to keep the baby in good position for birth.

When I discovered I was pregnant with my first child, I hired a licensed midwife and enjoyed receiving my prenatal care appointments in my home. There is nothing like taking care of your annual pap smear without having to leave your own bedroom! The pregnancy progressed normally without any complications and my due date came and went. Then the pregnancy kept on progressing and I had to go for a consultation with an OB after being more than a week overdue. To my chagrin, I learned that the baby was double footling breech and, while my cervix seemed ready for labor, the baby wasn't settling down into my pelvis. I tried to hide my extreme disappointment and scheduled a cesarean for the following

185

week, secretly hoping the baby might turn and I would go into labor beforehand. At home, I did what every other modern, well-educated mother-to-be might do: I Googled "how to turn a breech baby" and tried most of the seemingly safe home-remedies such as lying on a tilt board, using ice or music to stimulate the baby to wiggle around, and meditating, with no luck. In my case, it seemed a little late for moxibustion or homeopathy and even the OB couldn't turn the baby in her attempt at external version. It was about as hopeful as turning a frozen turkey inside its plastic wrapper.

You could say that I had the ideal cesarean birth. The medical team consisted of my favorite obstetrician, one of the fastest and most skilled anesthetists on this side of the Mississippi River, nurses who were my coworkers, and my best friend, who was the neonatal nurse practitioner providing care for my baby. I had haircuts that were more painful than the spinal anesthesia and my scar is so low I can wear even the tiniest bikini. Even my midwife was present and it was her first experience with cesarean birth. I got to hold my baby as soon as he turned pink. I guessed his weight exactly before they weighed him while I was being stitched up. When I got to my recovery room, my family and baby were waiting for me. I happily munched a donut and milkshake and attempted to nurse my son. I had a little trouble with some heavy bleeding due to a retained clot and I was given extra pain medication since the doctor had to press on my fresh wound to get it out so, during that time, my husband went with the baby to the nursery with my friend and family for him to get his first bath while I waited for the heavy sedation to wear off. I was up on my feet by late that night and was back to feeling pretty good by about three weeks postpartum.

Making the choice to have a cesarean was not an easy one for me. I had read most of the relevant research on the risks of breech delivery and the increased chance of needing an emergency cesarean with a double footling due to the likelihood of a cord prolapse. The problem was I had personal experience with breech birth as a normal and natural way to give birth. During my first year as a nurse, I had a discussion with one of the more experienced obstetricians on the techniques used to assist breech babies in being born—more out of curiosity than anything else. The funny thing was that, within a week after that conversation, a woman arrived to my unit in the middle of the night ready to deliver any minute. She had been laboring throughout the day and, when we went to examine her, we were surprised by a couple of very cute baby feet! We called the physician but she was definitely going to give birth before he arrived. So I assisted the baby using the technique described to me by the doctor and the baby was born healthy and the mother had only a small tear. One of the most difficult things for me to deal with was trying to believe in the research data and ignore what I had seen with my own eyes.

Soon after my delivery, I began to have waves of sadness and feelings of regret. I was grieving for the loss of an experience that I had hoped to have. One of the other things that was very disturbing was how people didn't really want to hear about how upsetting having to go through the surgery was for me. The typical response, "Well, it's what is best for the baby" did not make it any easier for me to feel good about it. I was able to put it out of my mind for a while, until my menstrual cycle returned. I think that the cramps reminded me of the pain after the surgery; and my return to fertility scared me somewhat because I did not want to have to face the feelings I had. None of my friends could relate to me because they all had seemingly perfect vaginal deliveries, even preferring forceps-assisted birth to having a cesarean. My mother and my husband did the best they could to listen to my feelings but they, too, could not totally relate to what I had gone through. I found some support online interacting with other cesarean moms who were troubled by having unwanted surgery. I probably could have used some therapy but it didn't occur to me at the time.

When I learned that I was pregnant with my daughter, I was determined to do whatever I could to prevent having another cesarean if possible. I hired another licensed midwife to provide my prenatal care. I ate a healthy diet and got plenty of rest. I sat on a birth ball regularly and always rested on my side with my belly leaning forward to encourage gravity to pull the baby into the head down position. When I was about 30 weeks along, one day I could tell the baby had turned breech because the hiccups were all the sudden in my ribs instead of my hip and I went home and did the hands and knees technique and she flipped right back into head down position. Phew! That day made me a little nervous.

I otherwise had no problems and, at seven months, went to the consultation appointment required for VBAC clients. The doctor counseled me on the risks of VBAC and filed my consent on my chart. Unfortunately, the next week I learned that the doctor had added that my VBAC "be performed only in a hospital" to my consultation letter and backed out of the relationship with my midwife because her hospital had banned VBAC deliveries. Now, I would have to deliver in a hospital and find a new provider late in my pregnancy. I found a Certified Nurse Midwife (CNM) with an OB supportive of VBACs, and made an appointment. During my appointment on my due date, I found out that my CNM had unexpectedly been let go from the practice because she had told the OB she was investigating the possibility of joining another group! So, again, I changed providers trying to have some consistency with the midwife I went to the new group and had to be counseled again by another physician. Unfortunately, (for me), my CNM got a couple days off since it was a holiday weekend and I got an OB I had never met at my VBAC delivery.

The best thing I ever did was hire my original licensed midwife to provide doula services since she wouldn't be able to provide the midwifery care. This not only gave me some continuity of care but also gave me someone I could trust to advocate for me when I planned to be experiencing the pains of labor. I started with contractions on Tuesday morning, early, around 3 a.m. They woke me up off and on but faded at 7 a.m. when my friend dropped off her children so I could babysit while she took her son to a medical procedure. She picked up her kids at noon and I was looking forward to lunch and a nap. I got the lunch but could not sleep because the contractions came back. I was supposed to go to the grocery store to get last minute items for the turkey dinner on Thursday. I knew Mom would be irritated if I didn't go get the gravy but something told me I didn't want to be in line and panting! So, I summoned my mom to come a day earlier than she was planning so she didn't have to drive overnight and I called my sister and told her to go to bed early.

I had contractions about every six minutes for several hours, and went ahead and got a nice hot shower at midnight, and did my hair and make-up since I couldn't sleep...and I knew there would be pictures! I would blow dry in between and squat with contractions. By 1:00 a.m., I was starting to really have to focus on relaxing during the contractions. So, I had my husband call the doula and my sister, who would make sure to take pictures. My general opinion is that labor is women's work. And, while husbands can be supportive, but it is best to also have another woman present. My husband seemed to appreciate having someone around who could guide him in supporting me. I joked with him that I hired her to boss him around while I was in too much pain to do it myself. My labor picked up and by about 7:00 a.m. we decided to go to the hospital since I had been about 3cm at 4:00 a.m.

When I arrived at the hospital, the admitting nurse lectured me about staying home too long and I had to tell her that coming to the hospital was plan B for me anyway and she should buzz off. Her monitor wasn't working right so I had to fix it for her in between contractions. I was still about 3 cms and the baby was further up and my contractions spaced out after arriving— probably due to the stress response negatively affecting the positive feedback loop of the contractions. By about 9:00 a.m., things were picking back up again and I had met the doctor and met my nurse for the day, and my friends (present at the previous birth) arrived. I had experienced back labor since the middle of the night but it suddenly went away around 11:00 a.m., most likely due to the baby changing positions. I got a little nervous when the doula got a call that one of her other clients was also in labor. She actually left for about an hour and a half to go for the delivery (thankfully one of her students was doing most of the work).

Sometime after my waters broke things got pretty intense and I was having a time not responding to the pressure and the urge to bear down. I was starting the transition stage and the nurse checked and I was 8cm, and starting to have some swelling. When I heard that I got pretty scared. I didn't think I could hold off long enough to reach full dilation and I knew that swelling can often prevent further dilation, so I decided I would try an epidural to help calm down. My friends argued with me for twenty minutes to make sure that was what I wanted because they new I wanted to have a natural childbirth. More importantly, I wanted to avoid a cesarean. I knew the anesthetist pretty well, and even managed to let out a little joke about how he talked slow so we could skip the consent part and go straight to putting it in! It worked pretty well and, two hours later, I was ready to push and that epidural was wearing off. Unfortunately during this time, I had developed a headache which was probably due to several factors, including sleep deprivation, lack of my usual cup of coffee, not eating much all day, and a bolus of IV fluids for the epidural. Every time I pushed, my head throbbed afterwards. That had to be the worst part.

My epidural had only been dosed for two hours, and had mostly worn off by time I was close to delivering. When I started pushing, I was complaining about the baby's foot pressing on my rib. When I was nearly done, I was letting off a few howls and at least one "perineal war cry" as the midwife would say. I had a small tear, which I certainly felt. I was a little surprised at how hard the last few pushes had to be to get the baby out. I don't regret the pain I felt at all and the sense of relief when my daughter was born was amazing. I couldn't believe how quickly it was over—and I was all done! No huge scar, no lying in bed for a day, no hobbling around for weeks. I was the happiest mom with a sore bottom in town. I was overcome with emotion just as I had been after my son's birth, but this time I felt connected to my child immediately. The doctor waited to cut the cord as I requested. I held and nursed my daughter for an hour and a half before releasing her to be weighed.

When she was born, nearly everyone in the room was in tears, even the doula and nurse. I was so happy to be able to have such a wonderful experience, and to share it with my husband, my son, my mother, my sister, my three closest friends, and even my brother and his fiancé. The doctor, also, seemed touched by the warmth in the room and she continued to round on me during my stay when the other on-call physician was supposed to see me. My VBAC birth was empowering and somewhat healing for me. I am so thankful for the support I received from my medical team and my doula.

JP is a wife and mother of two children. She currently works part time as a Neonatal Nurse Practitioner in a level 3 N.I.C.U. She enjoys the domestic arts of cooking, sewing, gardening, photography, and scrapbooking.

23. Don't Fix What Ain't Broken!
by Lauren Cooper

I'm not a cardiologist, but my heart beats just fine on its own without help. I'm not a pulmonologist, but I breathe just fine all of the time without being reminded or shown how. I'm not a gynecologist, but I ovulate on my own. And I think just fine on my own without a psychiatrist reminding me how. My stomach digests food on its own without being monitored by a gastroenterologist, and I even go to the bathroom on my own without being shown how, as well!

These are all normal functions that I do just fine on my own without the help of a doctor. Labor and birth are normal functions, too. My body doesn't need to be monitored or shown how to give birth; it's a natural process and it knows what to do.

Now, if I were having problems with, say, breathing or digestion, I'd go see a specialist for it, if necessary. Same thing with pregnancy and birth—if I have problems or concerns, I most certainly will consult with a specialist in that field. And by specialist in pregnancy and birth, I mean a midwife. An OB/GYN is trained in women's medicine in general, and if I have concerns over my or my baby's health during that time, I want a specialist, not just a general doctor who's actually trained as a surgeon and doesn't look at the process as a normal, naturally occurring process.

If I'm going to run a marathon or exercise, I'm not going to insist on doing it in a hospital "just in case." Do you do all of your exercising in a hospital? If you're an average, low-risk individual, I highly doubt it. Even if you're out of shape or have never exercised before, does that mean you're going to jog on the treadmill for the first time in the hospital, just to be sure that your body can actually do it? Probably not. You'd probably be more comfortable in your own home anyway, without being scrutinized and being told your body wasn't working efficiently enough. I know when I jog or exercise, I like to do it in my own house so that I don't have a bunch of strangers watching me. That's just me. It's my comfort zone. Same thing with birth. Just because you may not have done it before, or you may not do it every day, doesn't mean you can't do it. If anything, because it's not an every day occurrence for you, you're probably better off in the privacy of your own home with positive, encouraging support, and without strangers staring at you. I know when I'm jogging on my treadmill, no one in my house picks on me for how out of breath I get or tells me I need to run faster. I get to go at my own speed.

Now, will I have a midwife at my birth? Probably. But the difference between having a midwife at my house during my birth and going to a hospital and having a doctor for birth is this: at my house, I'm on my own turf. Midwives (generally) are supportive and encouraging to you and the natural process. They usually only intervene if there's a problem. Otherwise, most are just there to support. Can't say that for doctors and hospitals in most cases, can you? They want to monitor frequently, if not constantly, repeatedly poke and prod and check your cervix to assess if your body is working quickly enough for them or not. Doctors are in and out as they please, on their schedule. With a midwife at your house, you know right where they're at. They're there if you need them, and will usually leave you alone if that's what you want. At the hospital, even if you say "I want to be left alone," there's usually a doctor or a nurse knocking and coming in (if you're lucky enough to get someone who knocks first), flipping on the lights before asking, and interrupting your flow as they please.

When someone has a heart attack, we don't berate them with "You should have been at the hospital. You knew your heart was beating and therefore it could have stopped at any minute!" We all know and accept that sadly, quite often, these things are simply a part of life. So why is it that when something goes wrong during a birth, if that woman is not in a hospital, people come down on her like it's her fault for not being there?

I am so sick of people telling me I'm irresponsible or ignorant for planning a home birth next time. Do they think that home birth is a decision I've taken lightly without researching? Do they know that some studies have shown home birth to be SAFER than hospital delivery? I guess it's just hard for people to accept taking on responsibility for themselves and their children.

If "the doctor said to do this," then whatever the effect is, it's not their fault or doing; they weren't responsible for that action. Heaven forbid I actually make my own decisions and take responsibility. Many people are afraid of that. We aren't born afraid of giving birth—that fear is something we have been taught to feel, even though the instinct and knowledge of how to birth is inborn within us. Sometimes, we just need a little support in rediscovering what's been within us all along.

I've found that many of the people who are most opposed to my choices and insist on hospital deliveries are very religious. If God thought it was best and safest for his Son to be born without Mary being monitored, poked and prodded or in a hospital, then why is it irresponsible for me to want the same peace, privacy, and safety? I've also found that many gung-ho epidural proponents are ultra religious, too. If you are so religious and so faithful, why are you afraid of letting your body do what God designed it to do? Why are you trying to avoid the result of the original sin, where God said that because of that, He would make labor hard work for women? I may not be very religious, but I did grow up going to Church and to a Catholic school, and I just am so baffled at how people can say one thing and do something else that seems to go against their beliefs and their faith in God.

So, the next time anyone makes a comment like "You're not a doctor" or "You're putting yourself and your baby in danger! What if something happens?" I'll ask them if they went to the doctor last time they defecated or exercised, "just in case," or if they are scared because they're breathing and their heart is beating as we speak without being monitored by a doctor, and something could go wrong at any minute.

Don't "fix" what ain't broken!

Lauren Cooper's bio is in a preceding chapter.

24. I Didn't Know I Had That Kind of Strength
by Kathleen K.

When I found out I was pregnant, I knew I was going to have a Home-Birth After Cesarean (HBAC). We had moved about seven months before I became pregnant and, after we moved, I became friends with a wonderful group of naturally minded families. Gina (not her real name) was one of the women in this group who happened to be an underground midwife, so there was no question who we would have attend our birth. She herself had an Unassisted Birth After Cesarean (UBAC) around the time I was c-sectioned with my first baby. She was a Labor & Delivery nurse with the reputation that "her" patients didn't have c-sections. There was never any doubt from her or her assistants about my ability to VBAC so my husband and I were very confident and comfortable with her.

At my 40-week prenatal appointment, I requested a vaginal exam (the first of my pregnancy) just because I was curious. I was 1 cm dilated and 80% effaced, and "Peanut" was already at +2 station and firmly anterior. So, I was pretty darn happy. A week and several false alarms later, I was getting tired of waiting for this little kid to show up. We had actually called Gina twice, and we all thought it was "time," but after several hours of regular contractions, they would stop. I wasn't physically uncomfortable, just anxious to meet our baby. So, Joe and I had been trying to get labor going for about a week.

I started having contractions around 3:00 on Thursday the 7th of July (41 weeks exactly). But, I didn't really think too much about them. I wasn't timing or even paying really close attention...just sort of like, "Oh hey, there's another one." I helped my brother get some homework submitted for his online class, which had me distracted for a couple of hours and, after he left, I noticed I was still having them. Hmm...interesting. Joe got home from work around 5:00 and I told him I was having some "irritating-type" contractions...still quite manageable, but definitely noticeable. He, of course, started timing, and got a little irritated when I mentioned I may have had some leaky water about 3:30 or so. We called Gina around 5:30 and, after discussing it with her, decided it wasn't leaky water. I didn't want her to come until we were sure it was actual labor, so I told her we'd call her again if things didn't slow down. I laid on the couch, showered, walked, drank a lot of water, and sat on my birth ball to see if anything made the contractions stop. Joe was running around the house, finalizing the preparations, filling the tub, moving the food downstairs, and trying to time the contractions for me. It was pretty cute watching him run around all excited. Nothing made the contractions change, so we called Gina again around 8:30, and I told her I thought we were in labor and that I'd like her to come out.

She got to the house and I was sitting on the bed playing solitaire. She walked in and said, "Oh, so this is active labor?" She checked baby's position, listened to the heartbeat, and suggested we go for a brisk walk. So we all did...and it was definitely brisk. The contractions were annoying, but not anything I had to stop for. They picked up once we got home, and Joe and I cuddled in bed and he helped me relax through the stronger ones, while Gina read a book in the outer room. I remember getting hungry so I ate a bagel. I also discovered that if I were to go pee a lot, the contractions didn't seem so bad. About 11:30 p.m., Joe and I took another walk to see if it would get things moving more. When we got back, I was feeling pretty tired, so Joe and I laid down again and that's when I noticed the contractions were getting stronger, to the point where I had to pause in conversation for them. Joe was very good labor support here...rubbing my back and helping me relax with the Bradley Method techniques we practiced.

Around 12:30 a.m., I decided I wanted to get in the pool, and that felt incredible. It took the edge off the contractions beautifully. I still had to pause and breathe through them, but I was back to cracking jokes in between. Gina was particularly amused when I mentioned peeing in the pool and Joe got disgusted by the thought.

(Now here is where things get weird. Over the next 17 hours of laboring, I appeared to go through transition twice. Now, I never got a strong urge to push at those times, but it felt very good to push, so I went with it...won't make that mistake next time!)

I spent most of the night in the pool, with Joe in there with me. He was wonderful labor support, rubbing my back and my shoulders, and he and Gina poured water over my lower back during contractions...that was AWESOME!!

The first time I pushed, which was around 4:00 a.m. on Friday, I pushed for about an hour, then asked for a vaginal exam (the first of my labor) because I didn't feel like the baby was moving. Sure enough, I was only 5 cm. So I got out of the pool, took a shower, had a beer (which slowed things down and spaced things out), and napped between contractions for a couple of hours. I had some yogurt and Gina went home around 6:30 a.m. to get some sleep. While she was gone, Joe cooked me some breakfast, and my mother wondered what the heck was going on. She was upstairs babysitting our 21-month-old, Zack. When she saw Gina leave, she thought we had the baby. When Joe didn't say anything to her, she asked him, "Well, is it a girl or a boy?" He had to explain that we hadn't had the baby yet. At some point I got back in the pool, and labored there again. We called Gina to let her know I'd had some more bloody show (mucus plug) and things were getting harder to manage. So, she came back and we labored in the pool some more.

The second time it felt good to push was around 3:00 p.m. I did that for a half hour, didn't feel like baby was moving, and asked for another vaginal exam. I was only 6 cm and starting to swell a little. At this point, had I been in the hospital, I would have gotten an epidural. I was *so* incredibly tired and frustrated, and the contractions were incredibly intense. It took Joe on one side and Gina on the other, both pushing in a hip squeeze for it to do any good. I took another shower, had another beer (actually, I had the beer while in the shower), and tried to rest in bed again. (By the way, a beer in late labor doesn't do diddly-squat.) Gina suggested that I try to labor on the toilet or walk around to see if that helped. Now, this whole time, the only place I had any sort of relief was in the water, I DID NOT want to walk around or sit. I actually said, "I'm seriously considering going to the hospital just so I can get some rest." Gina gently reminded me that that would increase my risk of having another c-section, which I knew, but I didn't want to think about. We all thought we were looking at another REALLY long night of labor. She left again around 5:00 p.m. and I spent the next hour on all fours on the bed having incredibly intense contractions. I was absolutely miserable. Every contraction, I thought "epidural, epidural, epidural." Then I would think "c-section, c-section, c-section," then I would think "one more contraction, one more contraction, one more contraction." I took it one contraction at a time, and managed to make it through another hour.

At around 6:00 p.m., Joe forced (coerced, begged, and eventually ordered) me to take a walk outside with him. It took us 15 minutes to walk 500 feet. Every five steps, I had a contraction that doubled me over. Around 6:30 p.m., I got back into the pool and, after about two contractions, had the unmistakable, unbelievable, undeniable urge, and I mean URGE, to push. At this point, Joe sort of freaked out, which is understandable. He called Gina on her cell and told her I had to push. While he was calling her, I checked myself...an unusual experience may I say...and surprisingly, I knew what I was feeling...and what I was feeling was a baby's head, and cervix...CRAP...cervix...is that really cervix?. DAMMIT!! I'm STILL not complete. I told Joe there is still cervix there. Gina told him to tell me not to push. She was on her way.

So he got off the phone, and for the next half hour he alternated between begging and ordering me not to push. I wish we had it on tape, "Honey, don't push, you can't push. Honey, please, for me, DON'T PUSH. You're pushing, STOP IT!." I was actually biting on the side of the pool, and grabbing handfuls of his legs and clothes because I was trying so hard not to push. I couldn't help it, though, because, after a certain point, your body is going to do it anyway.

As much as Joe was trying to keep me from pushing, he also wouldn't let me check to see if I was complete yet. Every time I would reach down to check, he'd say, "Don't check. She's coming, she'll be here soon." He was very freaked out about the thought of having the baby without someone there, which I totally understand now. Then, I was a little annoyed. To a certain extent, I was nervous about checking, too, because if I wasn't complete, I was going to kill someone. Now, during the time when I wasn't allowed to push, he had my mom boil a big pot of water to heat up the pool. While I was climbing the walls during contractions, he kept asking me, "Can I go get the water now?" I can laugh about it now, but then I was really quite irritated at him for asking!

So about 7:40 or so, Joe called Gina and when he left the room I checked myself. HALLELUJAH! NO CERVIX!! He came back in, I told him I'm complete, and his face went white as a sheet. He said, "She says she's complete... Uh huh... Okay... Uh huh... Okay... Okay... Bye." Gina told him what to do over the phone so he was much calmer, "Don't pull on anything, keep baby under the water until it's all the way out, and go slow."

Once he had directions on what to do, he was fine...very calm and reassuring, and he just kept repeating those things to me while I pushed. In a brief flash of clarity, I told Joe to turn on the video camera, which I'm really glad for since we had no one to take pictures.

If you picture kneeling with your knees kind of far apart and then sitting back on your heels, that's how I was pushing. It only took a few pushes and I could feel the baby's head right at the opening. It was surreal to reach down and feel this little, fuzzy, hard thing there. I remember thinking, "That's not really that big." Little did I know how much bigger it would get!

I vocalized through all the pushing, mostly because I kept hearing Joe say "go slow", so I had a very sore throat the next morning. It was 38 minutes from when I started pushing until he was born. Gina happened to call back just as the full diameter of his head was crowning ("ring of fire" doesn't cover it), so she got to "hear" him being born. I was kind of in my own little world once the head came out. I remember looking down into the water, and watching this little dark shape come out, and seeing an ear. Gina told Joe to have me check around the neck for a cord, which there wasn't. It was a good thirty seconds until I had another contraction, so I just sat there feeling the head. It was incredible to feel an ear on this side, a nose over there, fuzzy hair...just incredible. I had another contraction, pushed really hard, and the whole body just slid out all at once, much faster than I expected. There was this second where time seemed to stand still for an instant and I looked down at this little body under the water and I didn't have one single thought in my head. You know in the movies where the scene freezes for an instant, but the character is still moving, and then the scene suddenly starts moving again? It was one of those.

I remember thinking "Oh my God." I picked him up and held him to my chest and rolled over on my side so I was leaning up against the side of the pool. I rubbed his back and he made some gurgly noises, and started mewling. It was a surprisingly peaceful moment, just letting his body do what it knew to. Joe told Gina, "We got baby" and I distinctly remember him giggling when baby started making noises. Gina asked him if the cord was "thumping" so I felt it (another surreal experience to feel the lifeline to your baby pulsing under your fingers), and said yes. She wanted to know how fast...which she told me later was the easiest way to measure the baby's pulse.

Joe put a towel over us and I asked him what time it was. Gina told him 8:18, since she knew we didn't have a clock. He talked to her for another minute or so (during which she says he was funny...very giddy...just like a first time dad). She told him to just have me hang out in the pool until she got there and then he hung up. We put a hat on baby and just took a few minutes to enjoy the moment. Then he asked me if he could go get the water, and I said fine, so he did, and the warm up of the water was wonderful. But, he managed to burn his hand emptying the pot into the pool.

When he went upstairs, he told mom, "We got a baby, but we don't know what it is yet."

My mom told me later, she thought, "How do you not know?" She didn't realize we just hadn't looked yet. After about ten minutes of staring in amazement at this new little baby, it finally occurred to me we didn't know if it was a girl or a boy, so we took a peek, and I said with a very shocked look on my face, "Oh my god, it's a boy!"

Joe giggled some more, and said, "Zack's got a brother!"

Eventually my mom came down and sat with me for awhile while Joe looked after Zack. After seeing me in the recovery room after the c-section, and in the pool after Dominic's birth, I hope she now has a better understanding of what childbirth is supposed to be, and why Zack's delivery was so awful for us.

I didn't expect the third stage contractions to be so strong. I was feeling them down my legs, just like the first stage ones, so that was pretty annoying. I also didn't expect my butt to be so sore. Someone I know once referred to birth as "shockingly rectal". I would have to agree!

Gina got back at 8:50 and I thought I would get out of the pool to push out the placenta, but I could feel his cord tugging a little bit when I moved so I said I thought it was too short to stand up. Joe cut the cord in the pool and Gina took the baby in a warm towel and handed him to Joe. Again, I thought I'd get out of the pool, but the contractions were still pretty strong so I decided to stay where I was. Two contractions later (I think) and I pushed out the placenta, which had to be the weirdest sensation ever! Gina scooped it up into an ice cream bucket and closed it up. I got out of the pool, got dried off, and into bed. Gina checked me out, and I had one incredibly superficial 1/4" tear, and some skid marks. Joe and I cuddled in bed with our new son while Gina cleaned everything up and started laundry. Mom got me a piece of Gramma's homemade lasagna, and we started calling family. Once everything was cleaned up, Gina pulled out the placenta bucket and showed it to us and explained the parts. She said he had a nice, thick cord and a good, strong sac. We finally got to sleep around 11:00 p.m. or so. What a long day!! Our new little boy was 8 pounds, 2 ounces and 21½ inches long.

When I think about it now, I know I would not have been psychologically able to labor in a hospital. I had a hard enough time with the memories of the c-section being at home. I have no doubt that if I had been in a hospital, I would have been sectioned again, probably about hour 18 or so. I seriously doubt I would have been "allowed" to go 28 hours for first

> *This birth doesn't fix or heal what I was put through during and after Zack's delivery. In fact, it makes me angrier about it since I now know what was taken away from us.*

stage. I think that, despite how much I wanted a natural childbirth, I would have caved to the epidural, which likely would have led to other interventions and eventually another surgery. Even if we had transferred so I could get pain relief and if I didn't wind up with surgery, I still would have regretted going in and getting the epidural. I would look back and wonder "Could I have done it without it?" Instead, I KNOW that I can and did. I didn't know I had that kind of strength. I'm so thankful that I had labor support who knew what I truly wanted, so when I was utterly exhausted and ready to give in, they didn't let me.

I also believe that we were meant to birth him unassisted. Gina had two assistants who could have been at the birth. When I went into labor, they were both out of town and unavailable. My dear friend, who was going to act as our doula, was out of state and unavailable. Another friend, who is also a doula and who offered to drive two hours to be with us, had a migraine and couldn't drive. That was the first migraine she's had in years. Having that many people who could have been there but were all unavailable is just too coincidental to ignore.

This birth doesn't fix or heal what I was put through during and after Zack's delivery. In fact, it makes me angrier about it since I now know what was taken away from us. I still have a lot of healing to do, but if I ever needed to know if I am strong enough to do something, I can look back at this birth and know that I am.

Kathleen K. lives in Illinois with her husband, Joe, and their two children, Zachary and Dominic. She was unnecessarily c-sectioned with her first son for breech presentation, which the doctors admitted later was done for liability reasons. She hopes to help improve the home birth climate in Illinois, and plans for any future children to be born at home.

25. To My Sweet Baby Logan Bob

by Emilie Jarman

Logan Phyllip, our third sweet boy, was born on July 1st of 2006. It was a beautiful, second VBAC that I had to fight tooth and nail for. My first son, Gavin, was delivered via c-section, and my second son, Nathan (Boobah), was a very difficult, painful, exhausting VBAC. After Gavin, I was so drugged up, I don't remember holding him for the first time, and the following days were pretty much a blur.

With Nathan, after 18 hours of labor and 3 hours of pushing that ended up in a forceps delivery, I was so exhausted and sick that the nurse gave me a shot and I passed out for five hours afterwards. I remember being so exhausted that it took some time to really bond with him.

Then comes Logan, a "surprise!" My husband was being discharged from the Army, we were moving from Alaska to Michigan, and I had just finished nursing school and wanted to start working, aside from the fact that I had a three-year-old and a one-year-old. When I found out that Logan was a boy, I knew I was going to be outnumbered in a big way!!!

I was induced one day before Logan's due date and the labor was just awesome...not so much the contractions, but the pushing, I just felt so connected to him, and I envisioned him moving down the birth canal, and actually felt him moving exactly how I envisioned it. Because of my husband being in the Army, we were alone for each of the boy's deliveries, but for Logan's birth, my mom, his mom, and his sister were there.

I pushed out that beautiful boy at 12:55 in the morning, a huge

9 pounds, 5 ounces, and with the biggest mitts I have ever seen! The second the doctor put him on my chest, I just cried and cried, I said, "Hi baby, look at those hands!" I fell head over heels immediately. I loved and cherished my last baby boy. He had lots of dark brown, fuzzy hair that stuck up all over his head, I loved that!! And I loved his big hands and feet so much. He was such a character; he just brought me pleasure and joy. With your third baby, you aren't so stressed out. And, you know how fast they grow up so you take special care to enjoy every second.

He was just, bottom line, a good, easy-to-please, happy baby. He started smiling at about three weeks and he had this huge, crooked, goofy little grin that people just raved about. He loved it when you would pat his hands down real fast and sing, "Logan Bob, Logan Bob, It's a baby Logan Bob." He would cheese at anyone who took even a second to flirt with him. When he was a couple of months old, he would try to chuckle but would just let out this adorable, loud squeak that of course delighted everyone. He was so loved by our families. He was the first grandbaby they actually got to spend any significant time with. And when he guzzled his bottle if I was on the phone or anything, they would just crack up because they could hear as he slurped and grunted and gulped like a baby piglet. And he still had that adorable hair. I called it his "cool dude Bob mohawk."

On September 23rd, Logan was very fussy; didn't wanna swing, didn't want to eat, didn't want to be held. My husband took him upstairs and I told him to put him on our bed, I thought it would be comfy for him and he might sleep a little better. Nathan played airplane with him, made him squeak, pushing his fat little hams up to his chest to make him grunt (weird, I know – it was his favorite game), and than laid him down to sleep. He walked away, but heard Logan cooing and came back and saw that he had kicked all of his blankets off, so he put him on his tummy, and then rubbed his back to sleep.

At 11:00, I sent my 15-year-old sister, Lucy, upstairs to get him because I knew he would probably be getting hungry soon. Never, never as long as I live will I forget her voice when she ran down the stairs, hysterical, screaming, "Emilie, he's not breathing!"

I ran up the stairs as fast as I could.....and then sank to my knees outside the bedroom door. My body literally, physically, gave out. Nathan rushed by me and ran into the room. When he picked him up, Logan let air out, and Nathan thought he was breathing and yelled, "He's okay." Then, of course, realized that he wasn't. He said to call 9-1-1, which my sister did, and I heard her screaming and crying, "The baby is not breathing!"

The next minutes were as close as I have ever been to losing my mind. I believe I was in some sort of primal, animal state, and I did absolutely nothing but stayed on my knees, screaming from the very depths of my soul. I could do nothing, nothing else but scream and pray. I promised God that if he brought Logan back I would devote mine and my children's lives to him, that I would never stray from him again.

I heard the sirens wailing down the street and the EMTs and police rushed into our house, and ran outside with him. My husband tried to get into the ambulance but they told him no. He came back in to get the keys, and I couldn't even compose myself to go with him. I couldn't move. I just prayed. And Lucy laid on the floor and prayed. Nathan's aunt lives next door to us and they heard me screaming, saw the ambulance, and came over.

Once I was able to get up, his cousin took me and my sister to the hospital, which is just three minutes down the road. On the way, I told everyone to please pray, pray, pray, pray, pray. My sister was sobbing and I told her she had to stop because I felt as though I was one hair away from going clinically insane. On the way, Nathan's cousin's girlfriend said that I couldn't think the worst, and I replied that I couldn't have any hope. I had to think the worst because I had to prepare myself. I think I knew in my heart that he wasn't coming back. I leaned on my sister and Crystal when we walked in and immediately got bombarded by the receptionist in my face, saying over and over, "We need your insurance information."

There was a policeman who needed to speak with me, and kept repeating his request to go into a side room. They were both up in my face and wouldn't give me any room to breathe. I finally screamed and punched the wall. The policeman yelled at me that this wasn't necessary, and told me to calm down. I asked him if he had children. He said yes, he did, but he would not behave that way.

Finally, my husband was with me. I don't know where he had been. He just appeared by my side and told them to leave me alone; he would answer any questions that they had. I asked him to please tell me if he thought Logan would be okay, what did he look like? My husband couldn't even answer me. He just cried and shrugged his shoulders and said they were working on him.

I sat there for 45 minutes with my sister and just prayed. The police spent half an hour interrogating my husband. I called my grandma and told her that God wouldn't listen to me, but to please pray, because I knew he would listen to her. This whole time I just tried to keep the panic away and pray.

Finally, the doctor and nurses came out and told us in front of everyone, "I'm sorry, he is not here anymore."

I couldn't contemplate that. Not here? Where? What? It was not real. They said they were able to get air into his lungs, but couldn't start his heart. I said nothing, I didn't cry, I just stared at the doctor in disbelief. My husband crumpled and started wailing. They took us into the family room and said that we couldn't see him until the medical examiner came. Nathan's aunt had called our families and my in-laws arrived, then my mom and dad.

I didn't want to see him; I just wanted to remember him the way he was. I was afraid that he would be blue or not look like my sweet Logan. My husband told me that I had to, though, and that he was not going to leave until I saw him. After the medical examiner came, we were given a private room, and they brought in the same rocking chair from the same room he was born in. They wrapped him up in warm blankets and laid him on the bed.

When I walked in, it just struck me that this wasn't real. He looked like he was sleeping!!! I knew he wasn't "not here anymore." We got to spend three hours with him, holding him, telling him we love him, crying. Nathan's parents and my parents and sisters all held him, and then we held him alone. My mom cut a locket of his sweet, silky hair. His face was getting bruised and he was starting to not look like our sweet Logan, and the nurses kept telling us the state police had to start their investigation and it was time. Our whole family was there and I wailed as I handed MY boy, MY baby, MY son to a nurse who promised me that she would keep him in her arms until the funeral home came to take him to the other hospital to get his state required autopsy.

At 4 a.m., I finally walked out of the hospital with empty arms, leaving my baby boy alone for the first time ever. Logan had a monkey, his little stuffed toy that made him squeak. I couldn't stand the thought of him being alone. Monkey did not leave Logan's side. We had Logan cremated and Monkey was with him. We could not stand the thought of him being alone in the cold, dark earth.

Logan was a special baby. Every parent says that about their child, and I believe that they are. But Logan...there was a reason that he was here, brought such a huge amount of joy, and then left so early. I don't know what the reason is but I do know this. I LOVE my baby boy, and I always will. And I will do everything in my power to prevent this from happening to another family. That is why I have shared this story.

All three of my boys slept on their tummies. I thought that Sudden Infant Death Syndrome (SIDS) was kind of a myth, and that babies were more comfortable on their tummies, I thought I was doing the right thing for us. SIDS is not entirely preventable, but there are many things you can do to reduce your baby's risk of dying from SIDS. The number one thing is to lay your baby on his or her back to sleep. If I would have done that, perhaps Logan would still be here.....maybe he would not. But, I will never know. And that is what has brought me here to spread Logan's story.

I know my story is hard to read and I thank you for reading it. Every single second of his life, and even his death, is very important to us, and Logan will always, always be loved and remembered.

~~~~~

To my sweet baby Logan Bob........we all love you forever and ever. I hope you have lots of Monkey Slippers to play with in heaven, and I wait for the day when we will be together. You are Mommy's sweet boy.

Index

Printed in the United States
97720LV00002B/152/A